Table of Contents

CHAPTER 8: 110
OTHER NUTRITION HOT TOPICS & MYTHS
- Does Keto really work? Will fasting harm or help? Is animal protein harmful? What about dairy, gluten, and sugar substitutes? Your path through the maze of today's hot nutrition topics and their controversial effects.

CHAPTER 9: 118
NAVIGATING YOUR JOURNEY FAQ'S
- Setting your diet up is just the beginning. With this easy to understand Q&A, learn how to measure progress, break plateaus, switch up goals, and gauge when it's time for a diet break.

CHAPTER 10: 134
RULES FOR A WINNING MINDSET
- Three simple rules to making *Flexible Dieting with macros* a lifestyle you enjoy forever!

CHAPTER 11: 141
RECIPES THAT FIT YOUR MACROS
- Over fifty high-protein, low-cal recipes you will LOVE that keep diet goals in reach

CHAPTER 12: 196
MACRO-FRIENDLY RESTAURANT GUIDE
- Over 500 macro-friendly meals from over fifty fast food and restaurant chains to keep you on track on the go!

ACKNOWLEDGMENTS 207

REFERENCES 208

Introduction

Whether this is your first jump into the diet pool, or you've been to ample rodeos on the subject, you probably picked up this book because you're lost in the sea of diet insanity. There are countless books and programs to choose from. Whether it's Paleo, Weight Watchers, Vegan, Keto, Atkins, or more, every successful weight loss approach comes with tedious strategies and rules – eat more whole foods, fewer junk foods, and consume fewer calories. The problem with most of these diets is they eliminate so many foods – you must wave a permanent goodbye to meats, sugars, carbs, and anything else the diet deems an enemy. As every person is different, this isn't the end-all be-all, so most of these diets are nearly impossible to stick with long enough to see results. While you may see some short-term gains (or losses), it won't help much with maintaining your overall success.

Before we get started, let's make sure this guide is right for you:

→ You're not an elite athlete – working out is not your job but you like to be active.
→ You want to get fit and stay fit as you age.
→ You want to feel strong, look lean, and show the world you work out!
→ You want to figure out the right diet to lose body fat and gain muscle without those hard-to-live-up-to extremes that can compromise your metabolism, hormones, and make you feel like total garbage.

Well, I have some great news! This guide is designed to help people just like you! This guide encompasses my approach towards nutrition, what many like to call Flexible Dieting. It offers the structure you need while promoting choice and autonomy in the real world! Even if you have a basic understanding of what foods are healthy, you might still struggle to understand what really works for you. Tracking calories, macros, and eating for your specific needs will solve the mystery. *Flexible Dieting* puts you in the driver seat of your nutrition so you can get lean, strong, and healthy, all while living a life you actually enjoy. Don't get me wrong, any "diet" requires restraint and limitations, but it should never feel like punishment. Trust me when I say you can and will maintain your goals without unnecessary rules and restrictions.

I've helped thousands of people leave behind depriving diet behaviors and nonsense food rules by adopting a macro-based, balanced eating approach. My guides and instructions have left them stronger, leaner and more confident than ever before.

Excited? So am I, so let's dig in!

Hi, I'm Breanne!

The complicated world of dieting and nutrition can leave you feeling staggered, overwhelmed, and unsure of where to start (how I felt when I started my transformation!). But guess what! I'm here to help! This guide will empower you to control your own nutrition, reach your physique goals, and maintain them long-term.

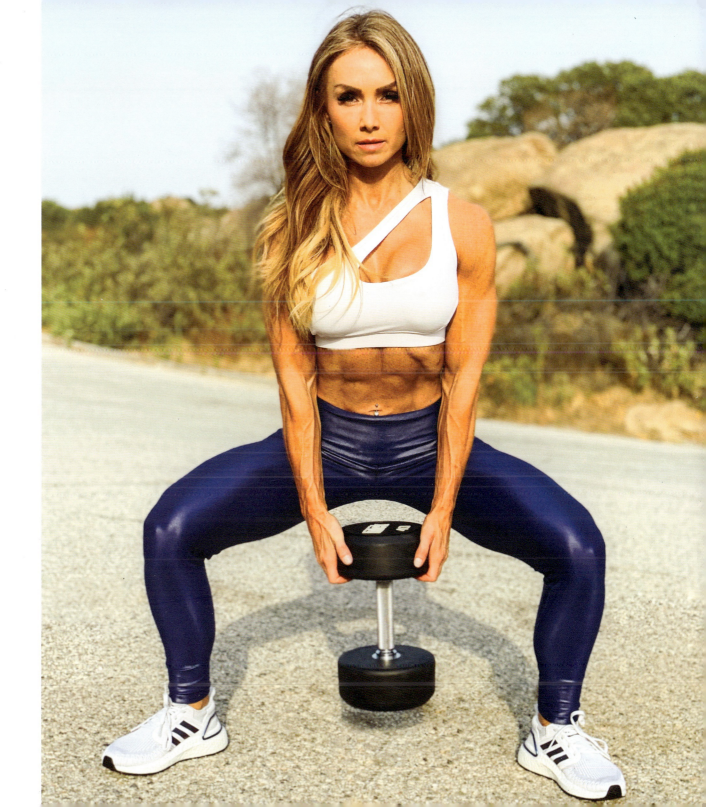

Table of Contents

INTRODUCTION 06

ABOUT BREANNE FREEMAN 07

ABBREVIATIONS & KEY TERMS 09

CHAPTER 1: 10
METABOLISM DE-MYSTIFIED
- Understand the various components of your metabolism and how to keep it firing.

CHAPTER 2: 19
THE DISH ON MACROS & MICROS
- Everything you need to know about protein, fat, carbs and micronutrients for optimizing your health and reaching your physique goals.

CHAPTER 3: 41
CALCULATE YOUR NUTRITION MASTER PLAN
- Discover what and how much you should eat to reach your goals.

CHAPTER 4: 56
CONQUER MACRO MEAL PLANNING
- Put your macro meal plan in place: what to prioritize, meal timing, macro cheat sheets, and my tried and true recipe-based 7-day meal plans.

CHAPTER 5: 78
FACTOR IN YOUR FUN
- Cheats, treats, travel, and alcohol – learn my tips and tricks for keeping favorites in your macro plan.

CHAPTER 6: 87
LET'S GET TRACKING
- Your step-by-step guide to tracking calories and macros with the *Lose It!* app.

CHAPTER 7: 99
SUPPLEMENTS WORTH TAKING
- Research-backed supplements to blast stubborn fat and build lean muscle.

About Breanne Freeman

My transformation is not your typical 'lost weight, got fit' story. I'm not someone who has ever been overweight or dealt with shedding pregnancy pounds. I started my fitness journey as an average girl who wanted to feel more confident in her skin. I had very little knowledge, however, of how to go about it. I visited the gym regularly, but never looked beyond group fitness classes, treadmills or ellipticals. I would indulge in McDonald's hamburgers one day, then starve myself the next. I didn't understand what a good fitness and nutrition plan looked like, and my body never changed because of it.

One day I was flipping through fitness magazines and I realized not everyone is built to be "skinny." I was 5'2" and already had a foundation of muscle built from my childhood years as a gymnast. It hit me! I needed to work with my body (not against it) to get the best results. I wanted to look strong like the women who graced these publications, but even though I continued to train HARD, I didn't look like it. I struggled with building muscle and chiseling fat. Something needed to change. So began my transformative journey, where I learned the proper art of weightlifting, a nutrition regimen, and the power within.

Years of studying evidence-based research, and a Nutrition Coach certification later, I can now look back and point out exactly which methods didn't align with my goals. The simple truth? Most of it had to do with nutrition. What we eat and drink has the largest influence over our results. Unfortunately, in our world of misinformation and fads, nutrition can be difficult to understand. That is why I wrote this guide. I want to share what I learned with you, and empower you with the knowledge to achieve your physique goals.

Success Story

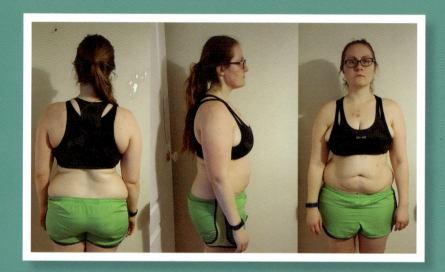 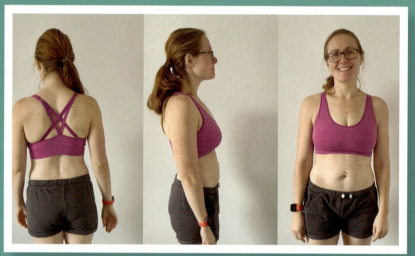

"If I can do it after three c-sections, a five, three, and one year old, then anyone can!"

I came from an active background, but three pregnancies and three c-sections took their toll on my body. Like most people, I didn't know where to begin. I was intimidated at the thought of counting macros, as that was something I thought only the serious dudes at the gym use. I was so wrong. Breanne's guide makes it simple and easy. The focus on lifting has been extremely beneficial as well. As a lifelong swimmer and runner, cardio used to be my mainstay, but adding lifting to my fitness regimen has caused greater changes in less time. Plus, I haven't run into the overuse injuries that used to plague me. Breanne's methods work, and if you are consistent and honest with yourself, you will be amazed at how your body can change.

In just 18 months, my body has transformed in ways I never dreamed possible. I dropped from 39% to 24% body fat and increased lean muscle mass from 34% to 43%. If I can do it after three c-sections, a five, three, and one year old, then anyone can!

I'm still not at my goal, but I have the tried-and-true tools to do it!

- Meghann Buckler

Abbreviations & Key Terms

1. **Macronutrients:** The nutrients our bodies use in big amounts to function properly including protein, carbs and fats.

2. **Micronutrients:** The nutrients our bodies need in smaller amounts to function properly. These include vitamins and minerals.

3. **Total Daily Energy Expenditure (TDEE):** the estimated calories your body needs to support your unique, day-to-day bodily functions.

4. **Basal Metabolic Rate (BMR):** the calories burned through basic bodily functions necessary for life: breathing, circulating blood, organ functions, and basic neurological functions.

5. **Thermic Effect of Food (TEF):** the calories spent to absorb, digest, store, and utilize the foods we eat.

6. **Exercise Activity Thermogenesis (EAT):** energy expended through sports-like activities and planned physical exercise and activities.

7. **Non-Exercise Activity Thermogenesis (NEAT):** energy expended for physical movement outside of sleeping, eating or sports-like exercise.

8. **Thermic Effect of Activity (TEA):** calorie use from day to day activity (NEAT), as well as planned/structured exercise (EAT).

9. **Muscle Protein Breakdown (MPB):** a naturally occurring process in which protein is lost as a result of exercise. If MPS outpaces MPB, muscle growth is achieved.

10. **Muscle Protein Synthesis (MPS):** a naturally occurring process in which protein is produced to repair muscle damage caused by intense exercise. It is an opposing force to muscle protein breakdown (MPB)

11. **Essential Amino Acid (EAA):** Nine amino acids the body cannot make, so you must get them through your diet. EAA's are vital for functions such as MPS, tissue repair and nutrient absorption.

12. **Branched Chain Amino Acid (BCAA):** Three of the nine EAA's mentioned above. These three compose 35% of EAA's in muscle proteins, and 40% of the preformed amino acids required by all mammals.

13. **Monounsaturated Fatty Acids (MUFA):** Unsaturated fats including olive oil, almonds, cashews, pecans; canola oil, avocados, olives, and nut butters like peanut or almond butter. All are an important part of a heart-healthy diet.

14. **Polyunsaturated Fatty Acids (PUFA):** Unsaturated fats including walnuts, sunflower seeds, flax oil, along with salmon and corn, soybean, and safflower oil which are an important part of a heart-healthy diet.

15. **Essential Fatty Acids (EFA):** Dietary fats Omega-3s and Omega-6s which cannot be synthesized by the body and must be consumed through food. EFA's are imperative to health and absorption of fat-soluble vitamins A, D, E, and K.

16. **Body Composition:** The proportion of body fat versus fat free mass within your body.

17. **Non-Nutritive Sweeteners (NNS):** A zero-calorie food additive that provides a sweet taste like that of sugar.

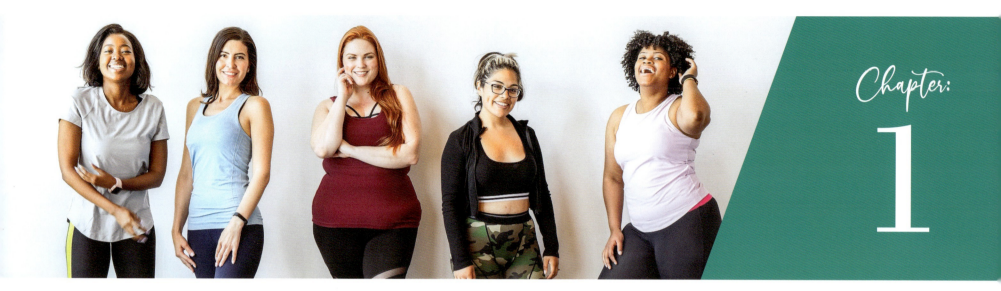

Metabolism De-mystified

A blanket approach to dieting doesn't work, and there's a lot of conflicting information out there that can mislead your daily decisions. Whether your goal is fat loss or muscle gain, you need a successful nutrition plan to support it. Let's start by taking the mystery out of how our metabolism works, and the way our bodies take in nutrition, process it, and use it to create energy. Simply put, that's called our energy balance.

Finding Your Energy Balance

The First law of Thermodynamics states that "energy cannot be created or destroyed, only transferred." No one is exempt from this law. What that means for us is that we take in energy in the form of calories from food and drinks, then we use that energy for daily bodily functions like standing, walking, breathing, eye movement, heartbeat, blood flow, fidgeting, digestion, formal exercise, and other physical activity. Your Total Daily Energy Expenditure (TDEE) is the estimated calories your body requires to support these functions every day. Energy balance means that when your calorie intake equals your TDEE, you will see no change in weight. If you eat fewer calories than your TDEE, you'll lose weight. If you eat more calories than your TDEE, you'll gain weight.

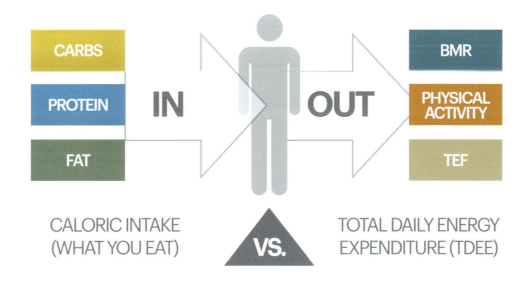

The number of calories in a food item is a measure of the potential energy that food possesses. There are three key macronutrients which make up the calories we consume in food: carbohydrates, protein, and fat. (Macronutrients are nutrients the body needs in large amounts.) One gram of carbohydrates has four calories, one gram of protein has four calories and one gram of fat has nine calories.

Various foods are a compilation of each macronutrient. If you know how many of each are present in any food item, you can calculate how many calories that food contains. Here is an example of a nutrition label. Don't be afraid of math! With a little practice, you can do this in your head while standing in the grocery aisle.

Nutrition Facts

Serving Size 1 bag (66g)
Serving Per Container 1

Amount Per Serving

Calories 240	Calories from Fat 72

% Daily Value*

Total Fat 8g	5%
Saturated Fat 1g	5%
Sodium 0 mg	0%
Total Carbohydrate 37g	11%
Dietary Fiber 6g	24%
Protein 5g	
Vitamin C 2%	Calcium 8%
Iron 30%	

*Percent Daily Values are based on a 2,000 calorie diet.

EQUATION

8g of Fat x 9 = 72 cals

37g of Carbs x 4 = 148 cals

5g of Protein x 4 = 20 cals

72 + 148 + 20 =
240 CALORIES

1g of Fat = 9 calories
1g of Protein = 4 calories
1g of Carbs = 4 calories

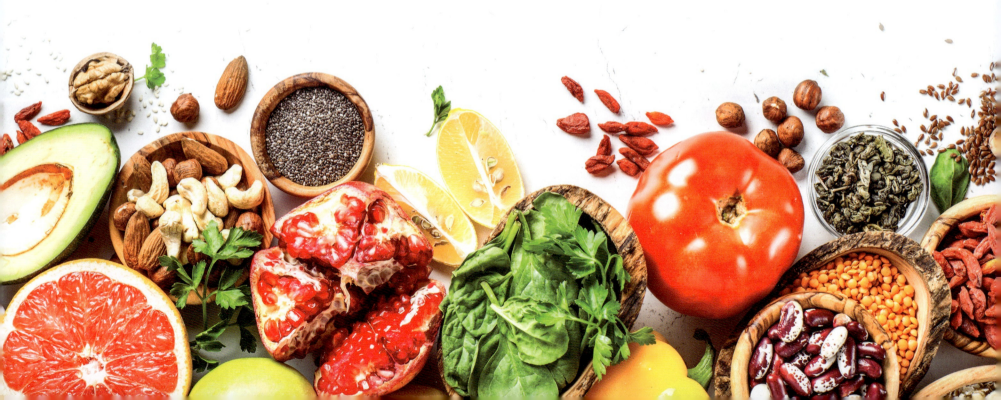

Solving Your Metabolism Mystery

Your Total Daily Energy Expenditure (TDEE) is your metabolism. When it comes to finding your energy balance, the 'calories out' side of the equation is not as simple as merely the number of calories you burn during formal exercise. How many calories you burn in a day can vary greatly from day to day and is unique to you.

We can estimate this calorie number by adding your body's baseline functions (BMR), your overall daily activity, and even the types of foods you consume (TEF). All variables are important truths to keep in mind when setting up your diet.

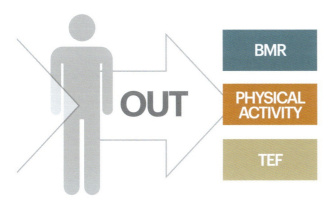

1. Basal Metabolic Rate (BMR)

Your BMR is the largest component of your metabolism. Essentially, it is the energy your body needs to survive at rest, and it accounts for 60-75% of your TDEE. For instance, as you read this your muscles are being used to hold your body upright in a seated position. Your eyes are reading the text, your brain is processing the information (and your brain uses lots of calories), your heart is beating, and you are breathing. All these body functions require calories. This is your BMR.

Various personal characteristics including body composition (fat vs. muscle mass), gender, age, height and weight also influence your BMR. In fact, your BMR is proportional to lean body mass and it has been shown to decrease relative to an increase in body fat mass [1]. Due to a variety of differences, your TDEE may not be comparable to someone else's of the same weight. For example, if you took two individuals of the same gender, age, height, and weight but one was 20% body fat and the other was 10% body fat, the leaner individual will most likely have a higher BMR and require more calories to maintain their weight.

Master Your Macros

It's also important to note that BMR declines with age, generally 2% and 3% per decade for men and women, mostly due to a loss in lean body mass [1]. Sarcopenia, or age-related muscle loss, begins around the age of 30 and increases after the age of 65. By the time you reach 65 up to 27% of your muscle mass could be lost [1].

Reduced physical activity, protein intake and anabolic hormones, like testosterone, are contributing factors to age related muscle loss. However, this can be minimized through consistency with a weight training regimen and proper diet, including sufficient protein intake. In the following pages, I will show you how to do just that.

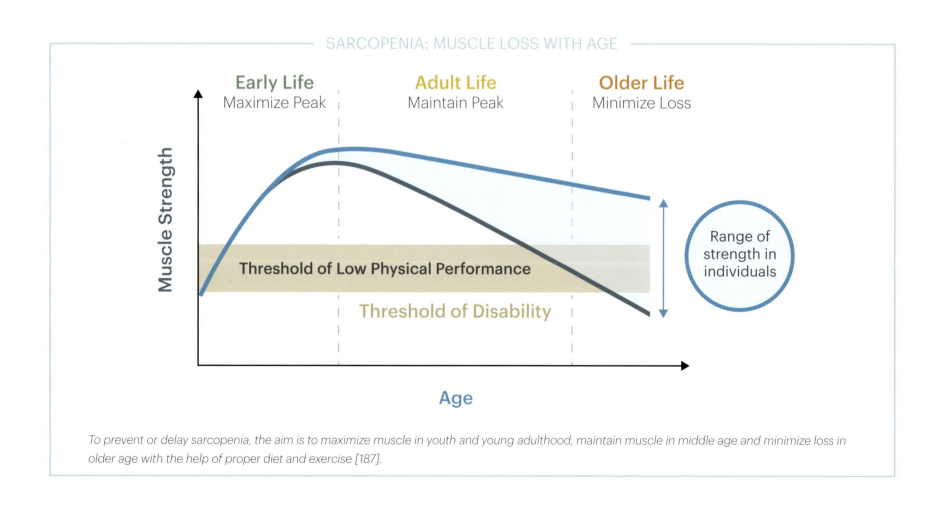

To prevent or delay sarcopenia, the aim is to maximize muscle in youth and young adulthood, maintain muscle in middle age and minimize loss in older age with the help of proper diet and exercise [187].

Master Your Macros

2. Thermic Effect of Food (TEF)

Just as each macronutrient (carbohydrates, fats or proteins) provides us with different calories per gram, they also require different amounts of energy to digest, absorb, utilize, and store. This process is called the Thermogenic Effect of Food (TEF) and accounts for around 10% of your TDEE. Yes, you are burning calories just by eating calories!

Research indicates the percentages of total calorie consumption to digest each macronutrient are: *0-3% for fat, 5-10% for carbohydrates, 20-35% for protein* [2,5].

Protein has the highest thermic effect and is also the most satiating macronutrient, leaving you feeling fuller longer than carbs or fat [3]. This is one of the many reasons why high protein diets typically result in greater fat loss and better improvements in body composition, even when caloric intake is equal. Likewise, complex carbohydrates, which are dense and higher in fiber, require more time and energy to be digested than simple carbohydrates do, also providing a more satiating effect. This isn't to say that any one food source is good or bad, they all play an important role within various contexts of your diet.

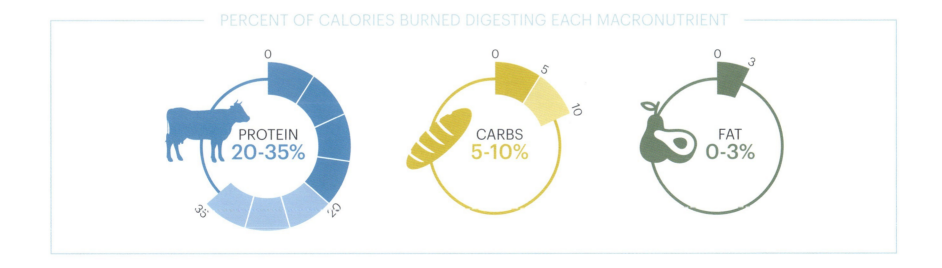

Master Your Macros

It's also important to note the effect processing has on food. This can impact how the food is digested and absorbed by the body which alters its thermogenic effect. When a meal of whole food and a meal of processed food are compared– meals of similar content, macronutrients, and calories– a 50% decrease in thermic effect was reported with the highly processed version [4]. A highly processed food usually means fiber, vitamins, and minerals have been removed, and typically, sugars have been added.

Altering digestive workload can also be as simple as eating ground beef vs. steak or peanut butter vs. peanuts. This doesn't make ground beef or peanut butter unhealthy. In fact, you're likely to actually absorb more of the nutrients and protein from foods like these than you would otherwise. Additionally, none of this is to say the processing of foods or ingredients is inherently bad. Food processing can improve some food quality, increase convenience, help people who struggle to eat enough, and make life more enjoyable often without significant health consequences. The key is selecting the right "processed" foods. It's also important to keep in mind the number of calories those processed foods represent.

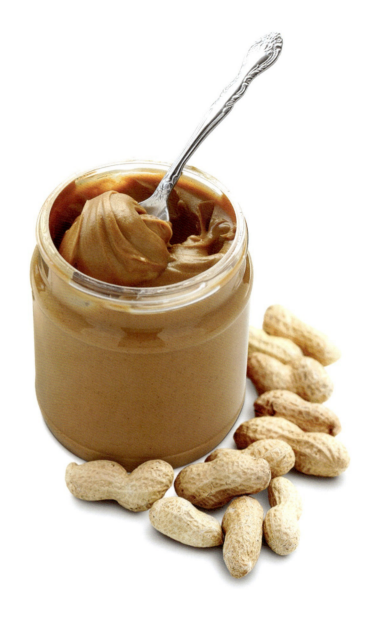

3. Thermic Effect of Activity (TEA)

The word "thermic" means heat, or in our case, energy expended. When using this word in relation to body functions, it means the energy we use to burn calories. When put together with the word "genesis" (meaning the beginning of something), it means the beginning of how we burn calories on a daily basis. The simple, non-exercise activities, thus Non-Exercise Activity Thermogenesis (NEAT) and formal exercise, or Exercise Activity Thermogenesis (EAT).

What you do each day–your TEA– accounts for 15-30% of your TDEE and will vary greatly between sedentary and active lifestyles. This component of metabolism is made up of two parts. The first part is NEAT, such as fidgeting, typing at your desk, grocery shopping, house cleaning, walking to and from your car, etc. The second part is EAT, such as jogging, biking, (basically any form of cardio), and weightlifting.

The importance of NEAT in your energy balance becomes more apparent when considering the BMR and TEF of individuals of the same gender, along with similar age and weight, is relatively fixed. BMR varies approximately 7-9% while TEF is maximally 15% [6]. Since exercise activity is believed to be negligible on a general population level, NEAT represents the most variable component of your TDEE. NEAT is responsible for 6-10% of the TDEE within sedentary lifestyles and up to 50% in highly active lifestyles [6]. If you have ever felt frustrated that your friend of the same sex, similar weight, age, and exercise regimen can eat more without fat gain, they likely have higher levels of daily NEAT.

If you have fat-loss goals, an effective strategy beyond exercise is to simply move more. Take daily walks, use the stairs instead of the elevator, park farther away from the grocery store, and fidget a little more. More movement throughout your day could result in up to 2,000 calories burned per day depending on body weight and level of activity [7].

Individual Metabolism Variations

So, now we know there are tremendous variations in rates of energy expenditure for all individuals. Some individuals that have a high BMR probably eat a diet that stimulates TEF, are very active, and have higher NEAT levels that likely cause them to burn calories at a faster rate than others.

In addition to variations in energy expenditure, there are also different rates of nutrient absorption between individuals as well. For example, if two people consume the exact same food, the total number of calories extracted, and the total amount of nutrients extracted can vary. Some foods require different enzymes to break them down, which may or may not be present in the digestive tract of all individuals. Food allergies, such as Celiac disease, and bacterial cells in the human gastrointestinal tract (GIT) influence the rate of digestion and metabolism. An imbalance of normal gut microbes can cause gastrointestinal conditions such as inflammatory bowel disease (IBD) and irritable bowel syndrome (IBS). Hormones, such as low or high thyroid, estrogen, and testosterone levels can also influence overall metabolic rates. Always refer to a medical doctor if a disease or syndrome is suspected.

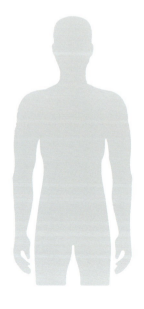

BODY COMPOSITION
Having a higher percentage of lean body weight creates a faster metabolic rate.

VERY LOW CALORIE DIETS
Eating behavior can alter your metabolic rate in adverse ways when you don't fuel your body sufficiently.

LIFESTYLE HABITS
A sedentary lifestyle leads to fewer calories burned.

CAFFEINE
Caffeine is believed to raise your metabolic rate.

HYPOTHYROIDISM
An underactive thyroid gland slows your metabolic rate.

AGE
As we age our lean body mass declines and we burn fewer calories. We also require fewercalories to sustain life.

BROWN FAT
If you are fortunate enough to be genetically blessed with a high percentage of brown fat then you likely burn calories a faster rate and have less storage adipose fat, but this is not something you can change through lifestyle.

FOOD ALLERGIES
Food allergies can lead to both weight loss and weight gain.

FOOD PROCESSING (THERMOGENESIS)
Digesting, absorbing, transporting and storing the food you consume also takes calories.

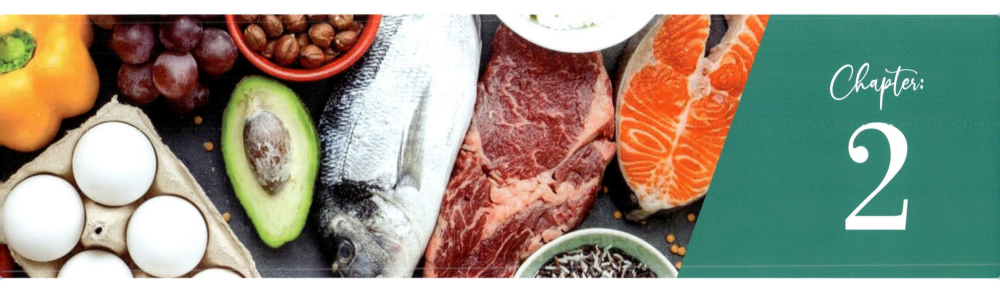

The Dish On Macros & Micros

There are three key macronutrients which make up the calories we consume in food. The prefix MACRO refers to the nutrients our bodies use in BIG amounts to function properly. These include protein, carbs, and fats.

The Power of Protein

I love protein, and for good reason! It is arguably the most important macronutrient. It's not a primary source of energy like carbs and fats, however, it is most often overlooked. Yet protein serves a much bigger purpose: it's the building block of our physical structure. It's what makes humans, well, human.
That body we're all looking for? It's all about protein!

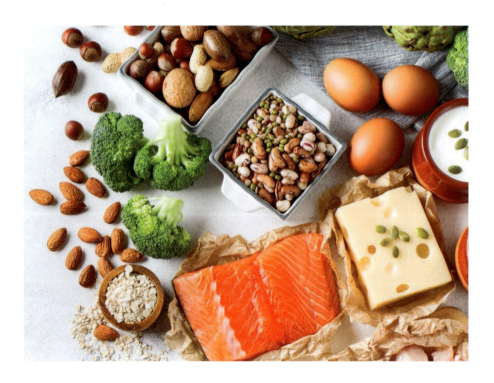

Why We Need Protein:

- It makes up the physical structure and growth of our body including our hair, skin, nails, bones, muscles, cartilage, and blood.

- It's used in nearly all bodily functions and processes including energy production, cell communication, fluid balance, pH balance, our immune system, and nutrient transport.

- Nearly all enzymes are made from protein. Enzymes are catalysts for chemical reactions in the body and are critical for many functions, particularly digestion and metabolism.

- Hormones that control hunger, satiation, physical growth, and repair are derived from protein like human growth hormone, insulin, gastrin, and leptin.

What's the Buzz About Protein?

I'm sure you've heard the saying "you are what you eat." In the case of protein, this is quite true! With the exception of water, protein is the second-most abundant molecule in non-fat bodily tissues, making up around 60% of our body mass. Then there's the rest of its impressive resume, listed in "Why We Need Protein" on page 20. Here's how it works:

Our body breaks the proteins we eat into amino acids. There are 20 amino acids required to support all our bodily functions. Nine of these are called Essential Amino Acids (EAA), meaning they cannot be made in the body and MUST be consumed through diet. Each of the nine EAA's have a unique job when it comes to keeping us strong and healthy:

>> **Lysine** plays a vital role in building muscle, maintaining bone strength, aiding recovery from injury or surgery, and regulating hormones, antibodies, and enzymes. It may also have antiviral effects.

>> **Histidine** facilitates growth, the creation of blood cells, and tissue repair. The body metabolizes histidine and histamine, which is crucial for immunity, reproductive health, and digestion. One study on obese women even suggested that histidine supplements may help lower BMI and insulin resistance [8].

>> **Threonine** is necessary for healthy skin and teeth, as it is a component in tooth enamel, collagen, and elastin. It also helps aid fat metabolism and may be beneficial for people with indigestion, anxiety, and mild depression. A 2018 study found that threonine deficiency led to a lowered resistance to disease [9].

>> **Methionine** plays a role in the health and flexibility of skin, hair and nails. It aids the proper absorption of selenium and zinc and the removal of heavy metals, such as lead and mercury.

>> **Valine** is essential for mental focus, muscle coordination and emotional calm. Deficiency may cause insomnia and reduced mental function.

>> **Isoleucine** helps with wound healing, immunity, blood sugar regulation, and hormone production. It is primarily present in muscle tissue and regulates energy levels. Older adults are more prone to isoleucine deficiency which may cause muscle wasting and shaking.

>> Leucine helps regulate blood sugar levels and is responsible for initiating the growth and repair of muscle and bone. It is also necessary for wound healing and the production of growth hormone. Leucine deficiency can lead to skin rashes, hair loss, and fatigue.

>> Phenylalanine helps the body use other amino acids as well as proteins and enzymes. The body converts phenylalanine to tyrosine, which is necessary for specific brain functions. Phenylalanine deficiency, though rare, can lead to poor weight gain in infants. It may also cause eczema, fatigue, and memory problems in adults.

>> Tryptophan is necessary for proper growth in infants and is a precursor of serotonin and melatonin. Serotonin is a neurotransmitter that regulates appetite, sleep, mood, and pain. Melatonin also regulates sleep. Tryptophan deficiency can cause a condition called pellagra, which can lead to dementia, skin rashes, and digestive issues. Studies have indicated that tryptophan supplementation can improve mental energy and emotional processing in healthy women [9,10].

Source: [11]

How Protein Helps You Reach Your Physique Goals

If you're reading this guide, you likely want to build muscle, burn fat, or a combo of both! Based on what we just learned about protein, I'm sure you can guess it's going to play an important role in helping you reach those goals.

When it comes to building muscle, the human body is in a constant state of flux. We are either breaking down muscle or building muscle. These activities are known as MPB (Muscle Protein Breakdown) and MPS (Muscle Protein Synthesis). We also know them, respectively, as catabolic and anabolic processes.

When an individual is gaining muscle and getting stronger, their body's rate of MPS is greater than MPB. Even if this individual is weight training regularly, without enough protein, it would be impossible to obtain the essential amino acids required to maintain and build this muscle tissue. This is particularly important for muscle retention on a fat-loss diet [12].

While some bodily functions require the help of a few EAA's, MPS requires that all nine EAA's be present, particularly valine, isoleucine, and leucine [10]. These three EAA's are known as Branched Chain Amino Acids (BCAA) and about half of the protein in your muscles is made from just those three [11]. Taking it a step further, you should also pay close attention to Leucine, which is the BCAA independently responsible for initiating the muscle building process. The amount of *Leucine* consumed in your food is the primary determinant of whether or not muscle growth occurs [12].

Protein also lends a big helping hand for your fat loss goals. First, as we learned in Chapter 1, protein is the most thermogenic macronutrient. This means you burn more calories just by digesting and processing protein than you do with carbs or fats. Second, sufficient protein intake helps you control your hunger in many ways. It digests slowly which helps you feel fuller for longer than if you consumed equal calories of carbs or fats [13]. It suppresses Ghrelin and Neuropeptide Y hormones, which stimulate hunger, while it increases GLP-1, Peptide YY, and cholecystokinin, the satiety hormones that stabilize blood sugar levels and help you feel full [14–19]. Third, sufficient protein intake helps preserve muscle mass, so the weight you're losing is mostly fat. From its muscle building properties to its ability to boost calorie burn, help us feel full, and reduce calorie intake, I think we can all agree that protein is the *super macronutrient* that will help you achieve that lean, strong physique you're aiming for.

BENEFITS OF HIGH PROTEIN DIETS

BETTER APPETITE CONTROL

Protein helps you feel satisfied and prevents hunger

METABOLIC BOOST

Protein helps burn more calories and prevents the slowing of metabolism that occurs when you lose weight

REDUCED FOOD CRAVINGS

Higher protein meals can help reduce cravings

IMPROVED BODY COMPOSITION

Higher protein diets results in greater fat loss and less muscle loss

REDUCED ENERGY INTAKE

Increases in protein at meals can have substaintial effects on energy intake, which is essential for weight loss

Animal vs. Plant-Based Proteins

All proteins are not created equal, and two things determine a protein's quality:

First is its *digestibility*. If you can't digest and absorb some of the protein you eat, then it may as well not have been eaten. Animal-based proteins consistently demonstrate a digestibility rate higher than 90%, whereas proteins from the best plant-based sources (legumes and grains) show a digestibility rate of 60–80% [20]. This is because plants contain anti-nutrients that inhibit protein digestion and absorption, meaning less of the plant-based protein you eat actually ends up in your blood [21]. While cooking does reduce anti-nutrient concentrations, it doesn't eliminate them entirely. It is possible to get the protein/amino acid combination you need, and I will address that in the coming pages.

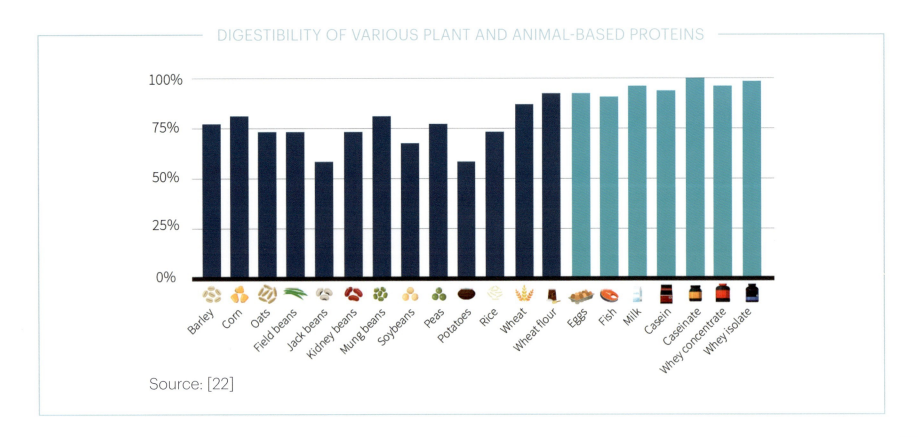

DIGESTIBILITY OF VARIOUS PLANT AND ANIMAL-BASED PROTEINS

Source: [22]

Master Your Macros

The second factor in a protein's quality is its *amino acid profile*. Remember, the right amino acids are extremely important if we want to build muscle. Different protein sources provide varying amounts and combinations of amino acids. Animal proteins are considered complete proteins because they contain all nine essential amino acids we need to build muscle, whereas many essential amino acids (EAA) are missing from plant-based proteins.

Leucine, the sole branch chain amino acid (BCAA) responsible for initiating the muscle building process, is the most common BCAA missing from plant proteins, followed by methionine, isoleucine, threonine and tryptophan. Lower leucine, and an essential amino acid profile of plant-based proteins, helps explain why several studies report lower rates of MPS from soy protein powders when compared to whey protein powders [23].

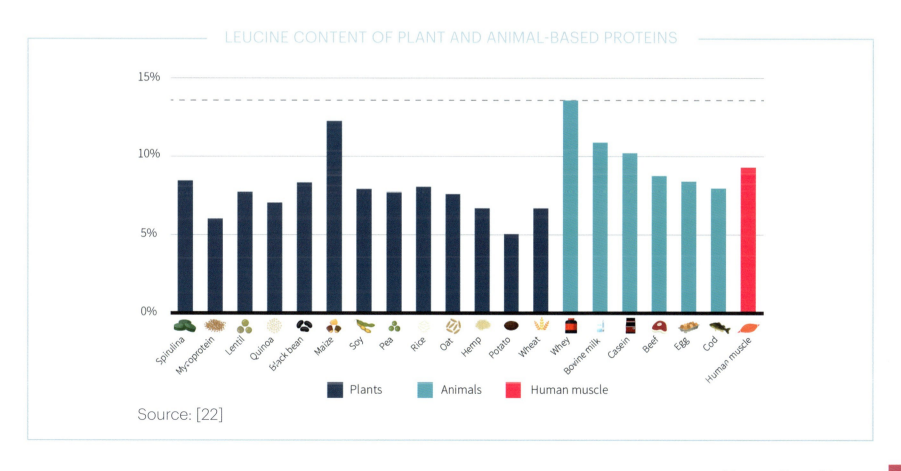

LEUCINE CONTENT OF PLANT AND ANIMAL-BASED PROTEINS

Source: [22]

For these two reasons, when following a plant-based diet, not only do you need to pay attention to the amount of protein you're eating, but also to the amino acid profile of that protein as well [24]. Plant based eaters typically need to eat more food and a larger variety of it to match the digestibility and essential amino acid (EAA) profile of animal proteins, especially when leucine is concerned.

This provides a challenge, and one potential solution is pairing two or more plant proteins to create a complete protein profile. Nuts and seeds tend to have lysine as a limiting amino acid. Beans and legumes, on the other hand, contain sufficient lysine but lack sulfurous amino acids, such as methionine and cysteine. Therefore, some great pairings would be rice + beans and pasta + peas, or whole wheat bread + peanut butter. There are a few plant protein sources with all EAA's. Soy tops the list with varieties like tofu, tempeh, and soymilk.

ESSENTIAL AMINO ACID CONTENT OF DIFFERENT FOODS

	Apples	Almonds	Rice	Beans	Tempeh	Dairy -2% Fat	Steak or Just Beef	Chicken
Histidine	✓	✓	✓	✓	✓	✓	✓	✓
Isoleucine	☐	✓	✓	✓	✓	✓	✓	✓
Leucine	✓	✓	✓	✓	✓	✓	✓	✓
Lysine	✓	☐	☐	✓	✓	✓	✓	✓
Methionine + Cysteine	☐	☐	✓	☐	✓	✓	✓	✓
Phenylalanine + Tyrosine	☐	✓	✓	✓	✓	✓	✓	✓
Threonine	☐	✓	✓	✓	✓	✓	✓	✓
Tryptophan	☐	✓	✓	✓	✓	✓	✓	✓
Valine	✓	✓	✓	✓	✓	✓	✓	✓

✓ Present at optimal levels   ☐ Not present at optimal levels

For example: One serving of rice (missing the EAA lysine) provides only four grams of protein. When paired with one serving of beans (missing the EAA methionine) you get an additional 13g of protein and all nine EAA's. It's important to note that while animal proteins are typically lean muscle tissue, plant protein sources typically contain additional carbohydrates and fat. The real challenge of relying on the rice and bean combo comes with the extra 70g of carbs and 280 calories to go along with it.

The good news is with the growing popularity of plant-based diets, many supplement companies have made large strides in improving high quality vegan protein powders — complimenting them with a full spectrum of essential amino acids. This is especially helpful for veggie-centric eaters trying to reduce calorie intake while keeping protein up. If eating plant-based is a non-negotiable for you, I highly recommend supplementing with a vegan protein blend that uses *rice* and *pea protein*. This blend is considered the "vegan whey", as it has a comparable amino acid profile to whey protein.

Optimal Protein Intake for Muscle Protein Synthesis

Regardless if you are a happy meat eater or dedicated herbivore, it's important to remember that small meals with limited protein, or proteins with low leucine content may be inadequate for muscle protein synthesis (MPS) to occur. It is estimated that you need around 2-3g of leucine, or up to 0.05g of leucine per kg of body weight to maximize MPS [25,26]. This is considered the leucine threshold. For example: If you weigh 125 pounds, 0.05g per kg of body weight requires about **2.5g of leucine** per meal to maximize the MPS response from that meal. Here are some examples:

Protein Source	Serving Weight	Total Calories
Whey Protein Isolate	23g	92
Soy Protein Isolate	31g	125
Skim Milk	374mL	333
Beef (raw weight)	142g	391
Chicken (raw weight)	142g	147
Peanuts	149g	876
Greek Yogurt	250g	143
Eggs (whole- large)	4.6 eggs	321

Collagen Considerations

As the desire grows for healthy, anti-aging benefits to improve skin, hair, and nail beauty, so too does the demand for collagen supplements. While numerous studies have reinforced these claims, collagen is much more than skin deep [27-29]. It also bolsters connective tissue, which supports your active muscles, and promotes the repair and the growth of new joint cartilage [27,30]. It improves bone mineral density and cardiovascular function [31]. Collagen supplementation can even lessen recovery time from athletic injury through its direct anti-inflammatory and antioxidant support [32]. One human study even found that 83% of the subjects had more energy and 70% reported that collagen improved their overall well-being [27,32]!

While there are clearly many benefits of adding collagen supplementation into your routine, it's important not to use it as a replacement for your whey or multi-source vegan proteins. Still, collagen provides a unique spectrum of amino acids; it's higher in glycine, proline and hydroxyproline, but lower in essential amino acids (EAA), especially tryptophan and leucine. As we learned above, complete protein sources with all EAA's are required for muscle growth, balancing blood sugar, keeping us fuller longer between meals, and fueling important metabolic functions [33].

To reap the benefits collagen has to offer, 10-15g per day is sufficient. It has also been found that Vitamin C plays a vital role in collagen synthesis, so combining these two is highly suggested [34]. Just make sure the rest of your protein comes from a variety of sources rich in all BCAA's with sufficient Leucine.

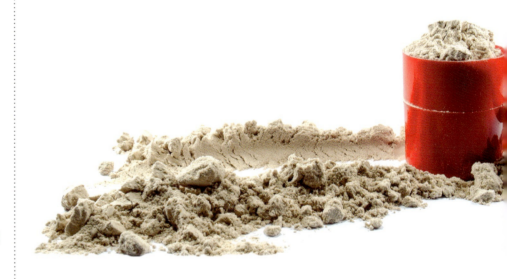

The Skinny on Fat

The word "fat" has gotten a bad rap. With two and one-half times more calories than protein and carbohydrates, fat is a major source of energy, but for decades, it was blamed for making us fat. Who remembers the plethora of fat-free foods that flooded grocery store shelves like Snackwells cookies and WOW chips in the 90's? In recent years, the pendulum has swung the other way. Trending diets are now calling for excessive fat intake, including buttery, oily cups of brewed coffee. What's a person to do?

Here's the deal: just like carbs, fat can be stored for later use as fat tissue. To get lean, strong, and optimize health, we should focus on consuming the right types and amounts of fats.

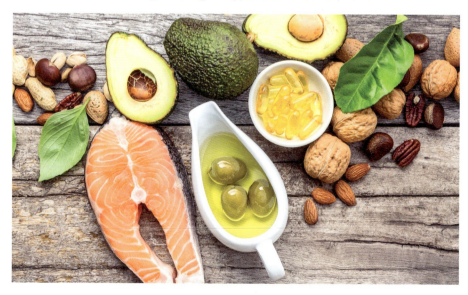

Why We Need Fats:

- Due to its high calorie content, fat provides a concentrated source of energy for the body.

- Fat is actively involved in healthy brain function.

- Maintaining healthy skin and hair can be helped with fat.

- It helps our body produce and balance hormones.

- Fat can help reduce inflammation and improve insulin sensitivity.

- Body fat itself helps regulate our body temperature and provide cushioning for our organs.

All Fats Are Not Equal

Fats have an important role in improving our overall health and well-being. They help us absorb and utilize fat-soluble vitamins A, D, E, & K. They are imperative for eye and brain development in a growing fetus, especially in the late stages of pregnancy [35]. There is evidence that eating high levels of healthy fats supports cognitive function, may lower levels of depression [36], and protect against Alzheimer's disease and dementia [37]. When it comes to our health and fitness goals, fats also help our bodies regulate the hormones that help with weight control and muscle building.

With all the benefits fats have to offer, factoring in the right types to your diet is important. Avocados, beef, and butter are all common sources of fat, but your selection of each makes all the difference between optimal health, obesity, and heart disease [21].

Saturated Fats
There are divided opinions whether saturated fats are harmful or beneficial. U.S. Dietary Guidelines recommend no more than 10% of total daily calories come from saturated fats [38]. These include:
- Those derived mainly from animal products including butter, cheese, beef, pork, chicken, full fat dairy, and egg yolks.
- Those derived from a few unique plant sources that also contain saturated fatty acids such as chocolate, cocoa butter, coconut and palm kernel oils.

Trans Fats
In 2015, this type of fat was determined to not be Generally Recognized as Safe (GRAS) by the FDA (Food and Drug Administration, 2018). Trans fats are:
- Artificial fats used that are used to extend the shelf life of processed foods.
- Certain condiments and snacks including margarine and vegetable shortening, fried foods, baked goods, processed treats, and non-dairy coffee creamer are common sources.
- Fats that adversely affect a range of cardiovascular disease risk factors, including raising low-density lipoproteins (LDLs) and triglycerides, lowering high-density lipoproteins (HDL), increasing inflammation, and promoting endothelial dysfunction [39].

Unsaturated Fats
Research shows that substituting unsaturated fats for saturated trans fats can significantly decrease a person's risk of cardiovascular disease [40]. Found primarily in vegetables and plant sources and categorized as monounsaturated (MUFA) or polyunsaturated (PUFA).

These beneficial fats include:
- Olive oil, almonds, cashews, peanuts, and pecans; canola oil, avocados, olives, peanut butter and almond butter.
- Walnuts, sunflower seeds, flax oil, salmon, or corn, soybean, and safflower oil.

In recent decades, there has been a greater understanding regarding the importance of consuming adequate amounts of dietary fat from plant-based unsaturated fats, particularly the **essential fatty acids** (EFA) omega-3 and omega-6. Omega-3 EFA is considered slightly more important, as the modern Western diet is likely to be more deficient in omega-3 than omega-6.

Where health and fitness goals are concerned, studies have shown some interesting findings with these fats.

Similar to protein, EFA's also trigger the release of the hormones GLP-1, Neuropeptide Y, and Cholecystokinin which reduce hunger and help you feel full [37,41-43]. Healthy fats can also improve insulin sensitivity which is particularly important for those with diabetes, prediabetes, fatty liver and elevated triglycerides [44-46]. Healthy fats have been linked to reduced inflammation and increased testosterone production, which may be beneficial for recovery from training, muscle building and fat-loss [47].

And so? Like I said, the word "fat" itself can throw people off, especially when looking at a nutrition label, restaurant menu items, and meal ingredients. Look for the good fats. They have your back, and every other part of you as well.

BENEFITS OF UNSATURATED FATS

HEART DISEASE PROTECTION

Consuming higher levels of unsaturated fats than saturated fats have a protective effect against heart disease

WEIGHT LOSS

Consuming unsaturated fats at meals can improve insulin sensitivity and feeling of satiety. A ratio of 1:5 saturated fats to unsaturated fats showed the highest occurrence of body fat loss

MUSCLE GAIN

Fat is the precursor for all-natural steroid hormones, including testosterone

MOOD BOOST

Replacing saturated fats with unsaturated fats can boost cognitive function and mood

Master Your Macros

The Carbohydrate Conundrum

All carbohydrates have one job: to give you energy. There is no 'essential carbohydrate' like essential amino acids from protein or essential fatty acids from fat, so you can technically survive without eating any carbs for the rest of your life. Trendy diets have many people drastically cutting carbs out of fear of gaining weight. In reality this does a disservice to your body and goals. Focusing on the right kinds of carbs will play an important role in providing the energy we need to maximize fat loss and muscle gain.

Why We Need Carbs:

- We need glucose to live and carbohydrates are our body's preferred glucose source.

- Our tissues, brain, and blood cells cannot make their own glucose, therefore we need an adequate intake of it.

- The brain is the largest consumer of glucose in the body [48]. When your brain seems foggy, low carbs are the likely culprit.

- Carbs optimize physical performance and post workout recovery.

- Many people don't know that fruits and vegetables are carbohydrates and they compose most of our micronutrients.

- Without carbs, we couldn't consume or process adequate fiber which provides numerous health benefits.

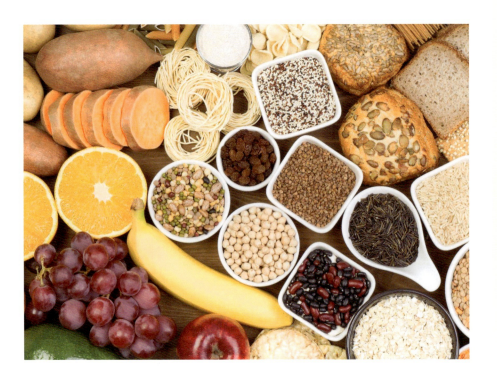

Carbs Fuel Our Fitness Goals

Like fat, carbs have gotten a bad rap over the years, but the truth is they're not the culprit for weight gain: it's a calorie surplus from all food sources. Utilizing the right kinds of carbs in our diet plays an important role in weight management and building muscle. Here are a few things you should know about these misunderstood macronutrients.

Burning body fat involves a carbohydrate byproduct. In situations of extreme calorie restrictions or inadequate carbohydrate intake, the body produces glucose (the body's storage form of carbohydrates) from non-carbohydrate sources, including amino acids taken from muscle tissue. Essentially, the body turns against itself through the "catabolization" (break down) of muscle tissue for the glucose it needs. Therefore, dietary intake of adequate amounts of carbohydrates can spare muscle tissue. One study published by the International Journal of Obesity compared the results of a high fat vs. high carbohydrate diet coupled with weight training over the course of seven weeks. The result: weight dropped in both groups, however body fat only decreased in the high carbohydrate group [49]. Thus, there is a clear distinction between weight loss and fat loss; carbs are quite important for retaining muscle and burning fat.

The largest storage of glucose is within the muscles and is exclusively reserved to fuel muscular work, from daily physical activity and formal exercise. Normal storage is approximately 6.8g per pound of muscle tissue. Considering how muscle comprises approximately 30% of a woman's mass and 40% of a man's mass, this averages somewhere between 250 and 600g in muscle tissue [40,50,51]. Plenty of research shows that when carbohydrates are restricted, and muscle glycogen stores are depleted, exercise and strength training performance are negatively impacted [52-55]. Eating sufficient carbohydrates provides the energy needed in order to progressively lift heavier weight, increase the intensity of your workouts, and therefore stimulate muscle protein synthesis.

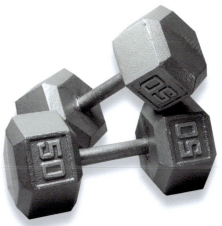

All Carbs Are Not Created Equal

Breads and pastas are carbs? Like fruits and vegetables? Well, yes and no. When looking at the entire carbohydrate family, bread, pasta, and potatoes look much different than milk, beans, fruit and vegetables. Just like fats, carbs contain a broad spectrum of foods with tons of misinformation to match. There's certainly room for confusion, but understanding the differences between these foods should help you prioritize the right carb sources in your diet. There are two types of carbohydrates: simple carbs and complex carbs.

Simple Carbs

- Smaller molecules of sugars the body breaks down easily to provide an immediate energy source.
- "Bad" Simple carbs generally come in processed foods like white bread, candy, cookies, soda, and fruit juices stripped of natural fiber and nutrients, while loaded with added sugars (cane sugar, brown sugar, honey, agave, coconut nectar, date sugar, turbinado, rice syrup, high fructose corn syrup, and many other aliases). These foods lack nutritional benefit beyond the immediate and very temporary energy boost they provide.
- Naturally occurring sugars are found in fruit, vegetables and milk. These are considered healthier options because they also provide important vitamins, minerals and fiber.
- Simple healthy carbs can be beneficial for pre-workout consumption as an immediate source of energy.
- US Dietary Guidelines recommend consuming 10% or less of calories from foods with added sugar, excluding fruit and milk [54]. Therefore, the less, the better.

Complex Carbs

- Contain a variety of vitamins, minerals and dietary fiber which take them longer to digest and provide energy over a greater period of time.
- These are often called "good" carbs, and for the most part they are found in their natural state like whole grains (bread, pasta, cereals), corn, rice, barley, quinoa, vegetables, beans, and wheat.
- These foods are key to long-term health. They make it easier to maintain a healthy weight and can even help guard against type 2 diabetes and cardiovascular problems in the future.

Fiber is Fabulous

Adequate intake of soluble and insoluble fibers provides many health benefits. These range from enhanced rates of weight loss and reduced cholesterol to improved digestive health and reduced risks of developing diabetes and cancer [59-61]. Therefore, we should strive to consume plenty of high-fiber foods. Most complex carbs that haven't been modified or processed contain all the nutrients the body needs for digestion and metabolism, particularly fiber.

Similar to protein, fiber plays an important role in fat loss by helping you control your hunger. First, dietary fiber is a less digestible carb, so it actually has different caloric values. Soluble fiber provides around two calories per gram and insoluble fiber provides close to zero calories per gram. This can also impact the absorption and alter the caloric implications of other foods eaten at the same time (one reason why calorie intake is not an exact science). Second, since it digests slowly, fiber helps keep you feeling fuller for longer than if you consumed equal calories of simple carbs. In fact, consumption of dietary fiber has shown to increase the hormones GLP-1, Peptide YY and Cholecystokinin which aid in stabilizing blood sugar levels and help you feel full [62–65].

Current *U.S. Dietary Guidelines recommend a daily fiber intake of 25g for women and 38g for men*. Keep in mind that excessive fiber can lead to bloating, poor nutrient absorption, and irregular bowel movements. Since current daily fiber intake averages around 18g per day for men and 15g per day for women [66], overconsumption is highly unlikely, but it is wise to introduce additional dietary fiber slowly over time to limit gastrointestinal issues and discomfort.

BENEFITS OF HIGH-FIBER DIETS

WEIGHT LOSS

Slower digestion delays gastric emptying to promote an overall feeling of fullness which can potentially reduce caloric intake

DIABETES PROTECTION

This carbohydrate is not absorbed and can reduce potential blood sugar spikes

INTESTINAL HEALTH

Fiber attracts water and it promotes bulk to the stool, which can safeguard against constipation

REDUCED CARDIOVASCULAR DISEASE RISK

Fiber can bind to cholesterol particles, prevent absorption, and help remove this compound from the body

[67]

Sugar Intake & Obesity Trends

A recent study on obesity rates and sugar intake should clear up some of the misunderstandings surrounding sugar. As obesity rates in the US continue to rise, added sugar intake has actually declined over the past 15 years [56]. In fact, on average, added sugars account for around 13% of total calorie intake in the US population. That's just 3% higher than US recommendations of 10%. Increases in obesity are therefore due to overconsumption of calories from ALL sources; not sugar by itself [57]. Still, it's a good idea to stay away from those carbonated drinks and snacks with lots of added sugars.

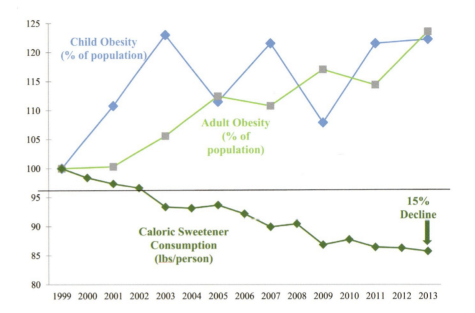

[58]

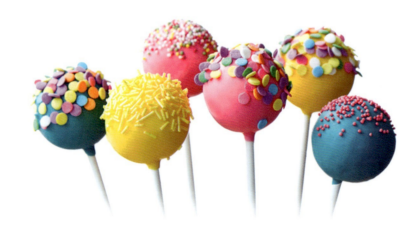

The Mighty Micro

Just as MACRO refers to the nutrients our bodies use in large amounts to function properly, MICROnutrients refer to those we need in smaller amounts. They are however, no less essential for optimal physical health and mental development. When you eat, you consume the vitamins that plants and animals created or the minerals they absorbed. Adequate intake of these vitamins and minerals is essential for optimal health, growth, immune function, brain development, energy metabolism, workout recovery, illness and disease prevention [68-71]. MICROnutrients are to humans as oil is to automobiles.

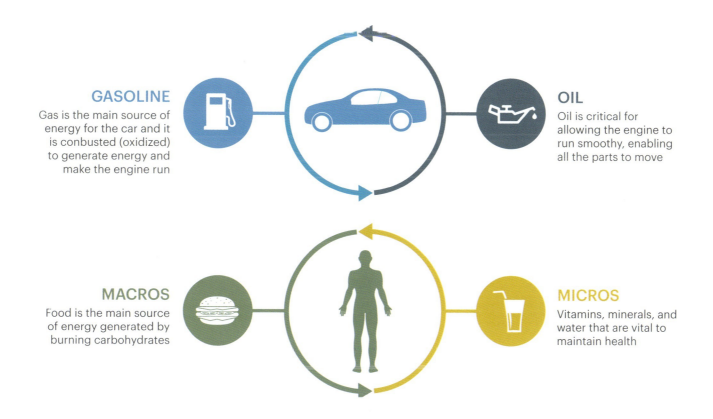

GASOLINE
Gas is the main source of energy for the car and it is conbusted (oxidized) to generate energy and make the engine run

OIL
Oil is critical for allowing the engine to run smoothy, enabling all the parts to move

MACROS
Food is the main source of energy generated by burning carbohydrates

MICROS
Vitamins, minerals, and water that are vital to maintain health

Micronutrient Deficiencies

Micronutrient deficiencies are rare in developed countries, but they do exist, nonetheless. Diets high in processed foods or those that eliminate major food groups are a major contributing factor to those deficiencies. Pregnant women and children under five have greater micronutrient needs. Symptoms of deficiencies include general fatigue, reduced ability to fight infections or impaired cognitive function including attention, concentration, focus, memory, and mood [72-74].

Achieving complete macro and micro-nutrition is nothing to worry about if you eat a well-balanced diet with several servings of fruits and vegetables, whole grains, lean meats, dairy and fish. It is best to avoid diets that promote severe restriction (very-low-carb diets for example), omit entire food groups (vegan diets or the keto diet), or follow very low calorie diets for extended periods of time. These can lead to large deficiencies in one or more micronutrients [75,76].

6 RULES FOR COMPLETE MICRONUTRITION

 01 80%+ of your diet should come from whole, minimally processed foods.

 04 Eat a wide variety of foods– think of the "rainbow" in fruits & vegetables.

 02 3-4 servings of green vegetables per day. 1 serving ~ 1 cup.

 05 Fatty fish 1-2 times per week, or take a fish oil supplement.

 03 2 servings of fruit per day. 1 serving ~ 80-150g raw weight.

 06 If grains, dairy or meat are eliminated: vitamin B12, vitamin D, iodine, iron, calcium, and zinc supplementation may be beneficial. Always consult with a medical professional.

Vitamin Cheat Sheet

Water Soluble Vitamins easily dissolve in water. They are not easily stored in your body and get flushed out with urine when consumed in excess.

B1
Helps convert food into energy.
Sources: whole grains, meat, fish.
RDI: 1.1–1.2mg*

B2
Necessary for energy production, cell function and fat metabolism.
Sources: organ meats, eggs, milk.
RDI: 1.1–1.3mg*

B3
Drives the production of energy from food.
Sources: meat, salmon, leafy greens, beans.
RDI: 14–16mg*

B5
Necessary for fatty acid synthesis.
Sources: organ meats, mushrooms, tuna, avocado.
RDI: 5mg*

B6
Helps your body release sugar from stored carbohydrates for energy and create red blood cells.
Sources: fish, milk, carrots, potatoes
RDI: 1.3mg*

B7
Plays a role in the metabolism of fatty acids, amino acids and glucose.
Sources: Eggs, almonds, spinach, sweet potatoes.
RDI: 30mcg*

B9
Important for proper cell division.
Sources: beef, liver, black-eyed peas, spinach, asparagus.
RDI: 400mg*

B12
Necessary for red blood cell formation and proper nervous system and brain function.
Sources: clams, fish, meat.
RDI: 2.4mcg*

C
Required for the creation of neurotransmitters and collagen, the main protein in your skin.
Sources: citrus fruits, bell peppers, brussels sprouts.
RDI: 75-90mg*

Fat Soluble Vitamins are best absorbed when consumed with a source of fat. They are stored in your liver and fatty tissues for future use.

A
Necessary for proper vision and organ function.
Sources: Retinol (liver, dairy, fish), Carotenoids (sweet potatoes, carrots.)
RDI: 700-900mcg*

D
Promotes proper immune function and assists in calcium absorption and bone growth.
Sources: Sunlight, fish oil, milk.
RDI: 600-800IU*

E
Assists immune function and acts as an antioxidant that protects cells from damage.
Sources: Sunflower seeds, wheat germ, almonds.
RDI: 15mg*

K
Required for blood clotting and proper bone development.
Sources: Leafy greens, soybeans, pumpkin.
RDI: 90-120mcg*

Master Your Macros

Mineral Cheat Sheet

Macro Minerals are needed in larger amounts in order to perform specific roles in your body.

CALCIUM
Necessary for proper structure and function of bones and teeth. Assists in muscle function and blood vessel contraction.
Sources: Milk products, leafy greens, broccoli.
RDI: 2,000–2,500mg*

MAGNESIUM
Assists with over 300 enzyme reactions, including regulation of blood pressure.
Sources: Almonds, cashews, black beans.
RDI: 310–420mg*

PHOSPHORUS
Part of bone and cell membrane structure.
Sources: Salmon, yogurt, turkey.
RDI: 700mg*

POTASSIUM
Electrolyte that maintains fluid status in cells and helps with nerve transmission and muscle function. **Sources:** Lentils, acorn squash, bananas.
RDI: 4,700mg*

SODIUM
Electrolyte that aids fluid balance and maintenance of blood pressure.
Sources: Salt, processed foods, canned soup.
RDI: 2,300mg*

CHLORIDE
Often found in combination with sodium. Helps maintain fluid balance and is used to make digestive juices.
Sources: Seaweed, salt, celery.
RDI: 1,800–2,300mg*

SULFUR
Part of every living tissue and contained in the amino acids methionine and cysteine. **Sources:** Garlic, onions, Brussels, eggs, mineral water.
RDI: None established

Trace Minerals needed in smaller amounts than macro-minerals, but still enable important functions in your body.

IRON
Helps provide oxygen to muscles and assists in the creation of certain hormones.
Sources: Oysters, white beans, spinach.
RDI: 8–18mg*

COPPER
Required for connective tissue formation, as well as normal brain and nervous system function.
Sources: Liver, crabs, cashews. **RDI:** 900mcg*

ZINC
Necessary for normal growth, immune function and wound healing.
Sources: Oysters, crab, chickpeas. **RDI:** 8–11mg*

MANGANESE
Assists in carbohydrate, amino acid and cholesterol metabolism.
Sources: Pineapple, pecans, peanuts.
RDI: 1.8-2.3mg*

Other trace minerals include: iodine, fluoride and selenium.

*Recommended Daily Intake (RDI) is for adults 19+ years of age in micrograms (mcg) in milligrams (mg) or International Units (IU). Source: [77]

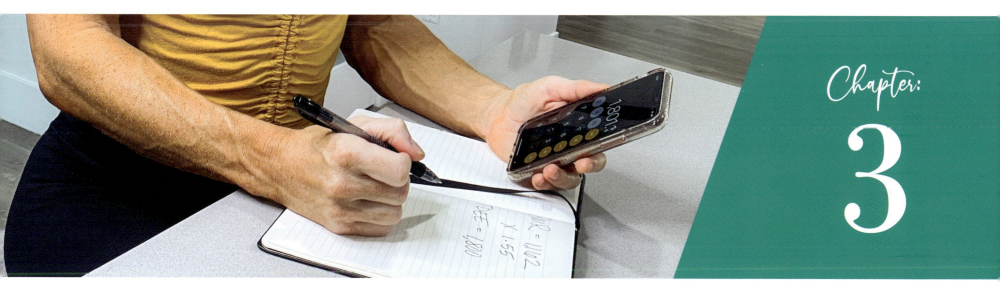

Calculate Your Macro Masterplan

Want to shed fat? Dream of building muscle? I wish I realized earlier in my journey that optimizing calorie and macronutrient intake for your goals is a powerful tool that can influence how hungry or full you feel, along with your metabolic rate, muscle building rate, and hormonal response [78]. Better late than never, right? So, it's time to whip out the calculator and get ready to find your personal macro masterplan.

What Fit & Healthy Looks Like

WOMEN

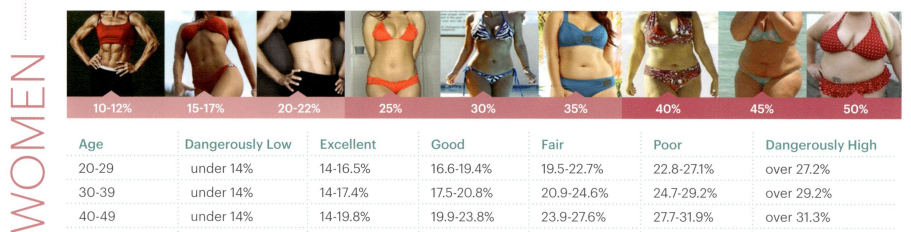

Age	Dangerously Low	Excellent	Good	Fair	Poor	Dangerously High
20-29	under 14%	14-16.5%	16.6-19.4%	19.5-22.7%	22.8-27.1%	over 27.2%
30-39	under 14%	14-17.4%	17.5-20.8%	20.9-24.6%	24.7-29.2%	over 29.2%
40-49	under 14%	14-19.8%	19.9-23.8%	23.9-27.6%	27.7-31.9%	over 31.3%
50-59	under 14%	14-22.5%	22.6-27%	27.1-30.4%	30.5-34.5%	over 34.6%
60+	under 14%	14-23.2%	23.3-27.9%	28-31.3%	31.4-35.4%	over 35.5%

MEN

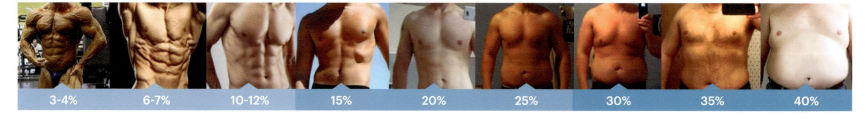

Age	Dangerously Low	Excellent	Good	Fair	Poor	Dangerously High
20-29	under 8%	8-10.5%	10.6-14.8%	14.9-18.6%	18.7-23.1%	over 23.2%
30-39	under 8%	8-14.5%	14.6-18.2%	18.3-21.3%	21.4-24.9%	over 25%
40-49	under 8%	8-17.4%	17.5-20.6%	20.7-23.4%	23.5-26.6%	over 26.7%
50-59	under 8%	8-19.1%	19.2-22.1%	22.2-24.6%	24.7-27.8%	over 27.9%
60+	under 8%	8-19.7%	19.8-22.6%	22.7-25.2%	25.3-28.4%	over 28.5%

Source: [79]

Understand Your Starting Point

Before planning the nutrition details of your physical transformation, it's helpful to gain understanding of your body composition, which is the proportion of fat mass to non-fat body mass, including muscle, bones, and organs. Knowing your body composition can help you assess your current health and fitness level. We've all got a "dream body" in our minds, but it's important to consider this:

Excessive body fat has been associated with coronary artery disease, hypertension, adult-onset diabetes, high cholesterol, obstructive pulmonary disease and osteoarthritis.

Too little body fat can affect fertility, immunity and disrupt heart health, sleep, energy levels, hunger, and stress. It also leads to serious physiological dysfunction [80].

Considering the health problems associated with too much or too little body fat, an assessment of your body composition can provide meaningful insights, while just scale weight or Body Mass Index (BMI) calculations make no distinction between water weight, lean muscle tissue, body fat, and bone mass. The images and tables on page 42 offer helpful guidelines. Acceptable ranges of fat mass slightly increase with age, and differences in hormones also mean women naturally carry up to two times more fat mass than men without additional health consequences. It's also important to know that two people with the same body fat percentage can look very different. Where we store fat and how quickly we build muscle depends mostly on genetics, but is also influenced by whether or not we regularly weight train and how consistent we are with a proper diet.

The rest of this chapter will guide you through choosing an appropriate goal and estimating your calorie and macronutrients targets to meet it.

How to Estimate Your Calorie Needs

1 **Choose Your Primary Goal: Blast Fat or Build Muscle**

Let's say you want to shed some body fat, but you also want to build muscle. Body recomposition, or building muscle while losing fat simultaneously, is the most sought after end-result. It's possible, and there are various circumstances it happens more often:

>> **Weight training beginners:** Your first one to two years of weight training is when your body responds and grows muscle the easiest, making faster recomposition possible.

>> **Detrained weight lifters:** If you've weight trained for years, but have recently taken a few months off, muscle memory ramps up muscle-protein synthesis (MPS) and makes recomposition possible.

>> **Overweight / Obese:** Those within poor or dangerously high body fat ranges easily have enough body fat to fuel the muscle building process while burning fat.

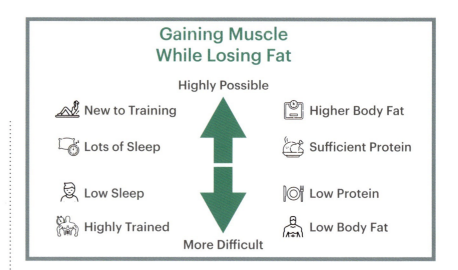

While some scenarios make body recomposition possible, if you want to do it well, the most practical approach is deciding what you want to achieve *first*, fat loss OR muscle gain, and following that plan until you've reached your desired outcome. Even if your training and nutrition supports a muscle gain plan, your metabolism will likely speed up as you gain muscle so you burn calories at a faster rate. Therefore, you could end up shedding some fat because of the muscle you've gained. Everybody will respond differently to a workout and nutrition regimen; we covered how this works in Chapter 1, Metabolism De-mystified.

If both objectives are equally important, a diet set up at-or close to-caloric maintenance (your TDEE) is ideal, but this can make results in either direction slow to achieve. I'll walk you through setting up your calorie and macronutrient intake next, but if you're undecided, consider these scenarios:

>> You are overweight: Even if you want to add muscle, it is likely more important for your health that you get leaner first. Those who are overweight and newer to weight training have an increased chance of building muscle while following a fat loss diet.

>> You are 'skinny fat': You're at a normal scale weight, but you have very little muscle and a relatively high body fat percentage. In this case, fat loss is likely a better goal for your physique and health. Those who are 'skinny fat' usually have very little weight training experience and therefore may add muscle as long as a weight training program is in place.

>> You have small problem areas: You're somewhat lean but 'problem areas' bother you (e.g. lower belly fat, hips and thighs, "love handles"). You also *really* want to add muscle. If those stubborn areas bother you the most, default to a slight calorie deficit for fat loss. If muscle gain is more important than those stubborn areas, shoot for maintenance calories or a slight calorie surplus for muscle gain. The closer you are to your maintenance calories on either spectrum, the more likely body recomposition can occur while following a properly programmed weight training regimen.

2. Estimate Your Total Daily Energy Expenditure (TDEE)

I'm going to give you some calculators here, ways to determine factors such as metabolic rates, calorie needs, and more. I know sometimes boxes of numbers can be scary, but trust me, it's a simple process!

Your TDEE is the estimated calories you need to maintain your current weight. You'll adjust from here based on your goal. There are also many online calculators to help estimate your BMR and TDEE. If you have tried any, you might have noticed slight differences in the results. This doesn't mean one calculator is more accurate than the other. They all just use equations generated from large population averages based on gender, age, height, and weight. Body composition is typically not accounted for, which is why these formulas are good, but not great.

How to Calculate Your TDEE

Determine Your BMR

Your Basal Metabolic Rate (BMR) is the number of calories it takes to support your metabolism at rest. The calculator found at http://www.bmrcalculator.org uses the Mifflin St. Jeor formula:

WOMEN BMR: [(10 x weight in kg)] + [(6.25 x height in cm)] − [(5 x age in years)] − 161 = [estimated calories burned at rest] ← This is your BMR.

MEN BMR: [(10 x weight in kg)] + [(6.25 x height in cm)] − [(5 x age in years)] + 5 = [estimated calories burned at rest] ← This is your BMR.

Determine Your TDEE

Your Total Daily Energy Expenditure (TDEE) is the number of calories it takes to support your BMR plus daily physical activity. To do this, multiply your BMR by your selected activity factor. Activity factors take into account your day-to-day movement and planned exercise. I recommend that you commit to one activity factor (don't think too hard about this!) and move on to the next step. There's always room to adjust calories down the road.

BMR X Activity Factor = [estimated calories burned per day] ← This is your Total Daily Energy Expenditure

Activity Factors:

1.2 — If you're sedentary, you work at a desk job and do very little exercise or housework.

1.55 — If you're moderately active, you're moving most of the day and/or exercise with a moderate to intense amount of effort 3-4 days of the week.

Most people will probably fall into this category - you work a sedentary job, but you train hard. Or, you train moderately, but you also have a job where you stand on your feet all the time.

1.375 — If you're mostly sedentary for work, but you do some walking, aerobic exercise and housework on most days of the week.

1.725 — If you're very active, you're vigorously exercising with a moderate to intense amount of effort 5-6 days per week or playing sports most days.

1.9 — If you're extra active, you're participating in vigorous exercise 6-7 days per week, such as a training athlete plus a job which requires physical exertion.

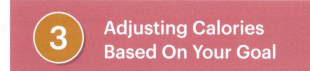

How to Adjust Calories for Fat Loss

Safe fat loss rates are typically 0.5% to 1% of your current body weight per week. When your primary goal is to lose fat, a calorie deficit below your TDEE is required. Fast rates of fat loss are motivating, but they are hard to sustain when hunger gets the best of you. Slow rates of fat loss are easier to sustain, but they also make it hard to stay motivated.

If you have a large amount of body fat to lose, I suggest shooting for 1% of your current body weight per week. If you're closing in on seeing your abs with less body fat to lose, you may err on the side of 0.5% loss per week, and sometimes lower if you're already VERY lean. Leaner individuals will find a slower approach to weight loss better for maximizing chances of holding onto muscle [81].

The theory says it takes a 3,500 calorie deficit for one pound of fat loss. For example, to lose 1/2 pound per week you need a 250 daily calorie deficit. To estimate the calories best suited for your fat loss goal, plug your numbers into the following equation.

How to Calculate Your Calorie Deficit:

Multiply your current body weight in pounds by your weight loss goal % per week (0.005 - 0.01) = _____ pounds per week loss.

Multiply that number x 3,500 (calories in 1 pound of body fat) = _____ calorie deficit per week.

Divide that number by 7 days in one week = _____ calorie deficit per day.

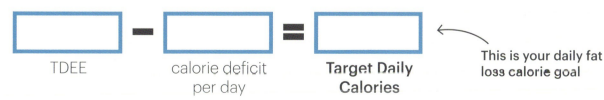

How to Adjust Calories for Muscle Gain

The goal of setting up a muscle building plan is to maximize the rate of muscle gain while minimizing unwanted weight gain. There are a lot of individual variables including age, weight training experience, body type, and genetics. **Remember:** an effective resistance program using progressive overload is also needed to provide the stimulus necessary for growth. Be patient and commit to your plan for a few months, since it needs time to be effective.

First, find your calorie surplus range:

Beginning Lifters: Those who have less than 2 years' experience. You can lift heavier & get stronger on a week to week basis and see significant visual changes month to month.	**TDEE to + 20%**
Intermediate Lifters: Those with 2-5 years' experience. You can lift heavier & get stronger on a month to month basis. Visual changes are evident every couple of months.	**TDEE to +15%**
Advanced Lifters: Those with 5+ years' experience. It takes months, even years, to see visual progress and the ability to lift heavier and make strength gains is very difficult.	**TDEE to +10%**

Next, identify your surplus target based on training experience:

• Is your current body fat percentage low? • Do you struggle to put on weight? Your body is more likely to use surplus calories for muscle gain	Go for a **larger calorie surplus** within your range.
• Is your current body fat percentage higher? • Do you put on weight easily? Your body can use stored fat to fuel the muscle building process + the more advanced you are the lower your surplus should be	Go for a **smaller calorie surplus** within your range, or even your **TDEE**.

How to Calculate Your Calorie Surplus:

TDEE x calorie surplus % (0.05 up to 0.2) = _____ calorie surplus per day.

[TDEE] + [calorie surplus per day] = [**Target Daily Calories**]

← This is your daily muscle gain calorie goal

Master Your Macros

Why Calorie Calculations Are Estimates

It's important to remember that hard numbers don't tell the whole story. I urge you not to over think the numbers you've calculated here. Calorie calculating isn't an exact science. BMR calculators and activity factors are equations and averages based on large populations. Your body composition, daily changes in Non-Exercise Activity Thermogenesis levels (NEAT), the variations in the thermic effect of the foods you eat (TEF), and various other metabolic factors make your TDEE, and therefore calorie requirements, unique to you. Additionally, when starting a diet, some may start to fidget or move less so NEAT levels might decline. No calorie calculation can take into account these differences so you will never know exactly how many calories you need per day. Consider this your starting point from which to adjust. Track your calories and macros after your initial calculation. Making refinements as your body responds is normal and essential. See Chapter 9, Navigating Your Journey for more information.

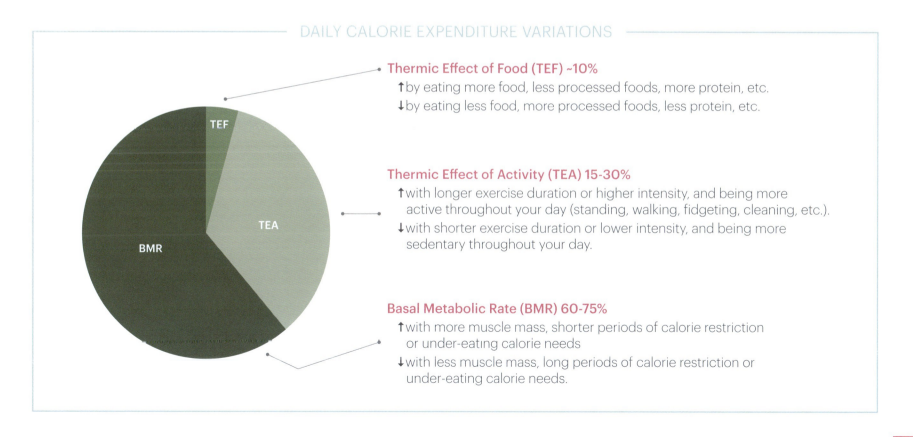

DAILY CALORIE EXPENDITURE VARIATIONS

Thermic Effect of Food (TEF) ~10%
- ↑ by eating more food, less processed foods, more protein, etc.
- ↓ by eating less food, more processed foods, less protein, etc.

Thermic Effect of Activity (TEA) 15-30%
- ↑ with longer exercise duration or higher intensity, and being more active throughout your day (standing, walking, fidgeting, cleaning, etc.).
- ↓ with shorter exercise duration or lower intensity, and being more sedentary throughout your day.

Basal Metabolic Rate (BMR) 60-75%
- ↑ with more muscle mass, shorter periods of calorie restriction or under-eating calorie needs
- ↓ with less muscle mass, long periods of calorie restriction or under-eating calorie needs.

How to Calculate Your Macros

PROTEIN

0.8g - 1g per pound you weigh everyday

Making this simple adjustment to my diet was game changing for my goals! What I want you to know there is a clear distinction between minimum daily protein requirements for basic health, and optimal intake to improve your rate of fat loss, muscle gain, and weight maintenance. Recent studies have even indicated the current Recommended Daily Allowance (RDA) of 0.8g of protein per kg of body weight per day has been underestimated up to 50% [82, 83]. Evidence shows daily intake of 0.8-1g of protein per pound (1.8-2.2g per kg) you weigh is optimal for muscle building as well as muscle preservation while dieting [33, 84, 85]. Intake up to 2g per pound you weigh everyday even appears to protect against fat gain while in a calorie surplus, especially when combined with resistance training [84,86]. Also, the older we get, the less efficient our bodies become at building muscle fromthe amino acids we eat, so those over 40 should err on the higher side [87].

Find your daily protein intake goal:

Are you trying to LOSE FAT and currently have a high body fat percentage? You are less likely to lose muscle in a calorie deficit	0.8g per pound you weigh
Are you trying to LOSE FAT and currently at a low body fat percentage? You are more likely to lose muscle in a calorie deficit	1g per pound you weigh
Are you trying to BUILD MUSCLE with a calorie surplus? Higher protein levels will protect against possible fat gain	1g per pound you weigh
Are you trying to MAINTAIN CURRENT WEIGHT at TDEE calorie intake	0.8g per pound you weigh
Are you 40+ YEARS OF AGE? Your body needs even more protein to support muscle building and preservation	1g per pound you weigh

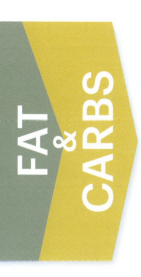

FAT & CARBS

20-35% daily calories from fat
Carbs fill remaining calories

Once you have your protein figured out, you can move on to your fat and carb goals. Neither are as black and white as protein intake. How much of each you should eat can vary based on body fat percentage, activity levels and even your eating preference. From a health perspective, it is recommended that 10% or less of calories come from saturated fats and trans fats to be avoided completely [38]. Stick to dietary fiber intake of 25g for women and 38g for men [55,88], while consuming 10% or less of calories from foods with added sugar, excluding fruit and milk [89].

Find your daily fat and carb intake goals:

Are you currently at a high body fat percentage?
Do you have a history of blood sugar regulation issues?
Do you suffer from hypoglycemia or hyperglycemia?
Do you have a sedentary desk job that takes up 30-50 hours of your average week?

30-35% calories from fat
Higher fat and lower carb intake may improve insulin sensitivity [90].

Are you currently at a low body fat percentage?
Do you participate in HIIT, endurance running, heavy weightlifting or strength training more often than steady-state cardio activity?

20-25% calories from fat
Higher carb intake may be best for performance and body composition [91].

Do you love fat-rich foods more than you love carbohydrate-rich foods?

30-35% calories from fat
More fats will make your nutrition plan more sustainable.

Do you love carbohydrate-rich foods more than you love fat-rich foods?
Do you prefer a plant-based diet?
You'll need to accommodate more carbs to reach your protein goal.

20-25% calories from fat
More carbs will make your nutrition plan more sustainable.

Master Your Macros

How to Calculate Your Macro Masterplan

PROTEIN

Determine Daily Protein Intake Goal. 1g of protein = 4 calories

_____ x _____ = ☐
(Current Body Weight) (0.8-1g / Day) **Daily Protein Goal in Grams**

_____ x 4 Calories = _____
(Daily Protein Goal) Daily Protein Calories

FAT

Determine Daily Fat Intake Goal. 1g of fat = 9 calories

_____ x _____ = _____
(Target Daily Calories) (0.20-0.35 from Fat %) Daily Fat Calories

_____ / 9 Calories = ☐
(Total Daily Fat Calories) **Daily Fat Goal in Grams**

CARBS

Determine Daily Carb Intake Goal. 1g of carbs = 4 calories

_____ - _____ = _____
(Target Daily Calories) (Calories from Protein + Fat) Daily Carb Calories

_____ / 4 Calories = ☐
(Daily Carb Calories) **Daily Carb Goal in Grams**

☐ = ☐ + ☐ + ☐
Target Daily Calories **Daily Protein Goal** **Daily Fat Goal** **Daily Carb Goal**

← This is your Macro Masterplan

Master Your Macros

Calorie & Macro Calculation Examples

WEIGHT LOSS:

Jennifer is 40 years, 5'4" and 154 pounds, 27% body fat and has a BMR of 1,356 calories. She wants to lose 1% body weight per week:

1. Moderate Exercise = 1,356 calories x 1.55 = 2,101 (TDEE).
2. 154 pounds x 1% = 1.5 pounds to lose each week.
3. 1.5 pounds x 3,500 = 5,250 weekly calories.
4. 5,250 / 7 = **750 daily weight loss calories.**
5. 2,101 (TDEE) - 750 = **1,351 daily calorie goal**

Protein = 154 pounds x 0.8g = 123g x 4 calories = 492 calories
Fat = 35% x 1,351 = 473 calories / 9 calories = 52g
Carbs = 386 calories left / 4 calories = 97g
Final Macros: 97g Carbs (29%) **123g Protein** (36%) **52g Fat** (35%)

See Jennifer's meal plan in Chapter 4

MUSCLE GAIN:

Stacy is 38 years, 5'5" and 127 pounds, 17% body fat and has a BMR of 1,250 calories. She wants to gain muscle and already has 6 years weightlifting experience:

1. Moderately Active: x 1.55 = 1,937 calories (TDEE)
2. 5% increase in calories: (TDEE) x .05 = **97 daily muscle gain calories**
3. 1,937 (TDEE) + 97 = **2,033 daily calorie goal**

Protein = 127 pounds x 1g = 127g x 4 calories = 508 calories
Fat = 25% (2,033) = 508 calories / 9 calories = 56g
Carbs = 1,017 calories left / 4 calories = 254g
Final Macros: 254g Carbs (50%) **127g Protein** (25%) **56g Fat** (25%)

See Stacy's meal plan in Chapter 4

Master Your Macros

Why Macronutrient Ratios Are Not Fixed

Contrary to what you might have heard, there is no ideal macronutrient ratio. Everyone will end up with a unique ratio of protein, carbs and fats depending on goals, calorie needs, body weight/composition and food preferences. While protein needs are fairly fixed and based on body weight, carb and fat ratios vary based on overall calorie needs. What's better is they can also fluctuate from day to day with no major impact on your health or goals. I think very little about the fats and carbs I'm eating as long as my calories and protein are in line with my plan. Not being fixed to a specific ratio allows for more flexibility in eating, more food variety, and better adherence to your diet plan. These examples are *only* provided to show you how your ratios may change as your goal changes.

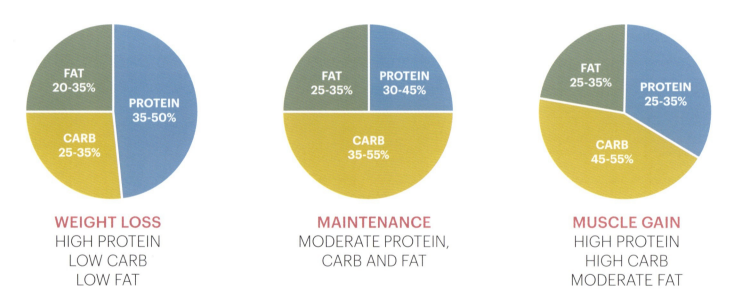

WEIGHT LOSS
HIGH PROTEIN
LOW CARB
LOW FAT

MAINTENANCE
MODERATE PROTEIN,
CARB AND FAT

MUSCLE GAIN
HIGH PROTEIN
HIGH CARB
MODERATE FAT

Chapter 9, "Navigating Your Journey," will help you understand if you set up your calories and macros correctly, when it's time to adjust, and answers to many other questions you may have as you navigate your body transformation journey.

Master Your Macros

Success Story

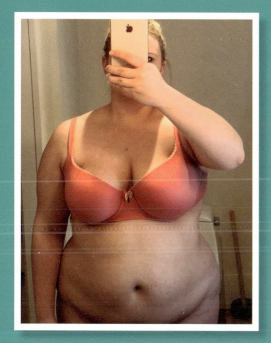
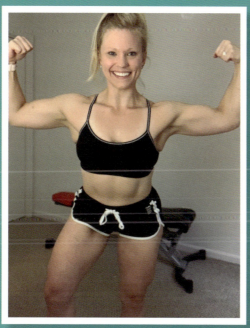

"I've gained 8.5 pounds of muscle, I'm leaner and feel more confident than ever!"

I was 24 when my doctor prescribed my first low-dose blood pressure medication. Years of binge drinking and closet eating finally caught up to me. My weight crept to 212 pounds, and plus size clothing was now my only option. Not only did I hate what I saw in the mirror, but my health was at serious risk. I needed to make some big changes.

The first 10 pounds fell off after cutting alcohol. My mind was finally clear, and I was to ready tackle a structured nutrition regimen. I was introduced to a plan that taught me about portion control. I learned a lot in just 6 weeks, but I craved more flexibility in my diet. I started a new plan that had me journaling everything–from food, to sleep, even bathroom habits. In seven months, 70 pounds were gone, and I was off blood pressure meds! I was proud of what I accomplished, but like a lot of people, I was stuck in a plateau for months and ready for the next step.

I found Breanne on social media and watched what she did for months. Her workouts, nutrition tips, and the physique she built intrigued me. Could I really build muscles like that without looking "bulky"? We seemed to be a similar height and build, so why not apply her nutrition and exercise recommendations and find out. To my surprise, I didn't have to adjust the foods I was eating by much. Her approach to nutrition, however, opened my eyes to the concept of fueling my body with intent. A simple adjustment to calories and protein intake is all it took to break my plateau and start seeing changes again.

> *I've been following this plan for a year now and the fat on my belly is continuing to melt, I've gained 8.5 pounds of muscle, I'm leaner and feel more confident than ever! The best part is none of this feels like a "diet," it's become a sustainable lifestyle I love!*

I've come a long way in just two years, but my journey is just getting started. I'm excited to see how my body will continue to grow and evolve. To have a physique like Breanne's, well I still have a way to go, but in the meantime, I'll be focused on tracking my macros, taking measurements, photos, and of course, lifting heavy!

- Kayla Rusiecki

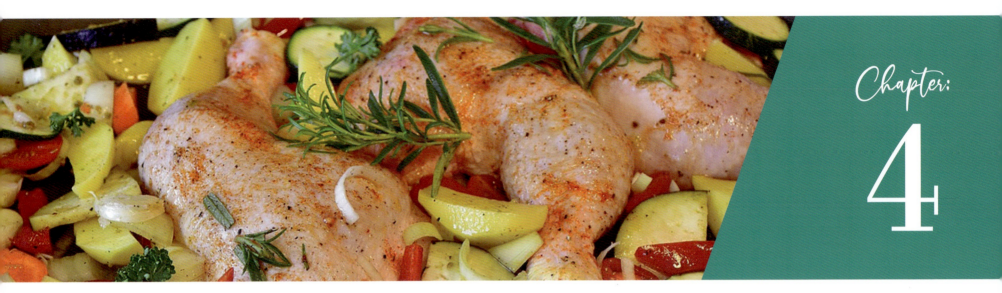

Chapter: 4

Conquer Macro Meal Planning

Now that you have a plan for what to eat to reach your goals, it's time to put your meal plan together. I've outlined my best tips and tricks to becoming a successful macro meal planner. You can also reference my macro cheat sheets and meal plans that have been designed using a variety of my tasty, high-protein recipes to get started.

What is Flexible Dieting?

Flexible Dieting is the beautiful intersection of eating for health and for enjoyment. It's a prescribed set of calories and macronutrients tailored to your unique needs (your macro master plan was just calculated in Chapter 3). At least 80% of your weekly calories is comprised of nutrient-dense, whole-food sources. It's the other 20% 'flexible' calories that are especially important because your quality of life and enjoyment in the process matters! A donut or slice of pizza every now an then is ok. Once I factored my favorite foods into my plan, I developed a healthier relationship with food. And those intense feelings of deprivation that failed me following other diet protocols are now non-existent. More flexibility with food choices increases dietary consistency, and consistency is the magic pill for reaching your goals!

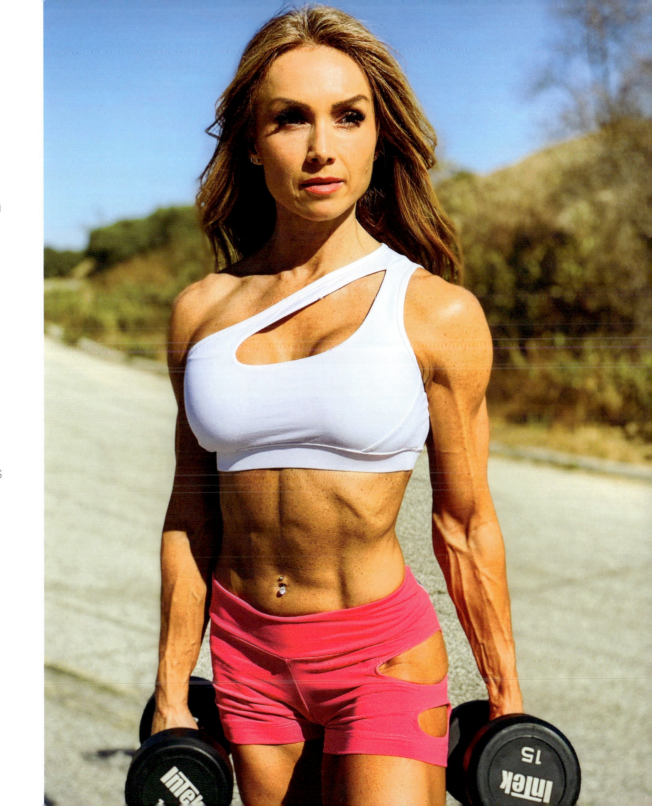

What You Should Prioritize

There are five main pillars of your nutrition plan and lifestyle that will have the biggest impact on your goals. Long-term *consistency* with all of these factors is critical in order to reach and maintain your results.

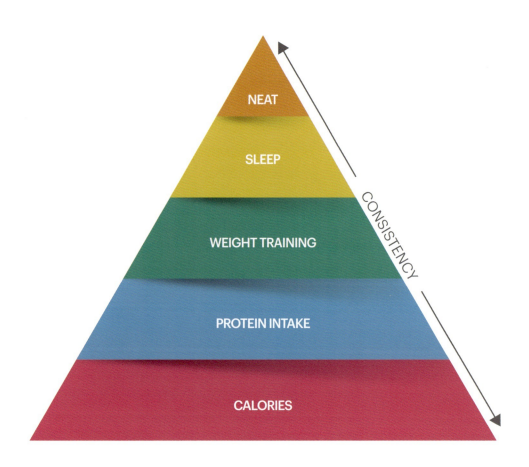

Jumpstart Your Macro Journey

Some meal plans can be intimidating and tedious, with massive, hard-to-track charts and way too much math. But there is an easier way, and I've got a few helpful hints to get you started.

 DOWNLOAD A FOOD TRACKER APP & START LOGGING YOUR MEALS

Before taking on your new nutrition plan, I highly suggest taking a week to track the food you currently eat in a calorie and macro tracking app like *Lose It!* Food tracking bridged my gap from macro-confused to macro-confident. Trust me when I say it's a much simpler and helpful tool than most people realize. *I have included a great tutorial for you in Chapter 6.* When you track every meal, snack, beverage and bite, **the calorie and macro calculations are done for you**!

 COMPARE YOUR CURRENT EATING HABITS WITH YOUR GOAL

Knowing how your current eating habits compare to the goal you just calculated is a great starting point. How far away is your calorie goal? How about Protein, Carbs and Fats? In my experience, many fall short on protein and tend to overeat carbs or fat. Even if only small adjustments are needed, tracking your food intake will be a huge help as you navigate your body's transformation journey.

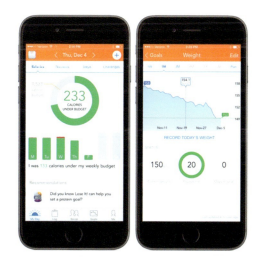

YOUR CALORIE & PROTEIN TARGETS ARE FIRST PRIORITY

You might have loads of macro targets to hit, and I know it can feel like piecing a puzzle together to reach your goals each day. Here's the thing, when it comes to changing your body composition, calories and protein will have the largest impact on your end result. As you gain confidence with tracking, your goal is to stay within 100 calories and 10g of your daily protein goal. As we have learned here, a good balance of fats and carbs are great for optimizing health and performance, but these two can vary more from day to day without compromising your results. Use your calculations as your guide, and if you feel and perform better with more fats and less carbs or vice versa, then that's ok. No matter what, don't stress over perfection, because it rarely exists.

 ### BE CONSISTENT

Calorie and macro tracking is a skill you develop over time and with practice. The more consistently and accurately you track, the more data you have about your eating pattern, and how it supports your goals, energy, and performance. Remember, no one starts as an expert – not in the kitchen, not while riding a bike, and certainly not here. The trick is to *just get started* and practice a little bit each day. Tracking your food will help guide you as you navigate your physique transformation journey:

>> Be Aware: Your calculations will show you how your typical foods and meals you eat impact your typical nutrition numbers. For example: nuts and avocado are healthy, but also very calorie dense. Taking in an extra 500 calories a day by nibbling on nuts all day makes consistently hitting your fat loss calorie targets difficult.

>> Be Accountable: If you aren't making progress and only hitting your target number, say 80% of the time, your calculations will reflect why. Changing your body composition requires consistency with your nutrition plan.

>> Get Educated: As we covered in Chapter 1, there are multiple variables that impact your energy balance. Using a calorie calculator provides a great starting point, but it isn't an exact science. Use this opportunity to learn about your body and its actual energy needs.

>> Develop Better Behaviors: The practice of tracking isn't always about the calories and macros. You won't lose weight and get stronger just because you meticulously count your calories and macros. Instead it draws sharp attention to the food you eat and can help with making healthier decisions. Calorie counting and food logging is one simple behavior that will inspire many other positive behaviors on your journey.

SELF-ASSESS AFTER 4 WEEKS

There is absolutely no reason, other than sickness or injury, to dramatically switch up your calorie and macro goals before four to six weeks of starting them, especially if they are improving the way you look, feel and perform. Knowing when to change a program requires adherence, along with other variables that impact your progress. So before switching things up, see how many variables you can check off the list to the right.

If you can check every box, and not seeing results, it's probably time to change things up. If you missed any, work on dialing those in over the next four weeks and reassess.

> Chapter 9, 'Navigating Your Journey,' will help you gauge the correct set up of calories and macros, how to measure progress, when it's time to adjust, and provide answers to many other important questions about your body transformation journey.

Nutrition Check List

- [ ] I have been accurately tracking my food
- [ ] I have adhered to my calorie and macro targets for at least four weeks
- [ ] I have tracked every bite or taste of food
- [ ] I have been eating mostly nutrient-dense foods
- [ ] I have been on track on weekends
- [ ] I have been tracking alcohol
- [ ] I have been weighing my food because it provides for better accuracy.

Training & Lifestyle Check List

- [ ] My workout program is tailored to my goal
- [ ] I have been consistent with my workouts
- [ ] I am training with progressive overload
- [ ] I am taking my rest days
- [ ] I am getting 7-8 hours of sleep (most nights)
- [ ] I am in control of my stress

Build Your Macro Meal Plan

Cooking healthy, delicious meals is a vital component for reaching your goals. It's important your meals fit within your daily target calorie goal, with appropriate quantities of protein, carbs, and fat. But meals should also taste good and be enjoyable to eat. Here are my best tips that keep goals in reach and your cravings satisfied.

 1. BREAK-UP YOUR CALORIE & MACRO GOALS INTO MEALS

I have found one way to combat the macro puzzle is dividing the number of meals and snacks you plan to eat whether it is three, four, or even six meals per day. This provides an idea how many calories, protein, carbs, and fats can be included in each meal. How many meals and snacks you eat depends on your total daily calorie budget and eating preference. For an individual whose calorie needs are below 1,500: three meals + one snack that is 150-200 calories will ensure the meals are larger and more satisfying. Those with calorie ranges of 1,500-1,800 per day: three meals + one to two snacks at 150-200 calories each is a good goal. If your calories needs are 1,800+, you may not find it comfortable or practical to eat just three meals a day because of the amount of food that needs to be consumed. In this case, consider splitting your meals into three to four meals + one to two snacks– the choice is always yours. You can even set your specific calorie and macro meal goals in the *Lose It!* app. Once you log your actual meals, *Lose It!* will recalculate the rest of your days' calorie and macro targets so you can stay on track at all times.

For an example, Stacy's muscle gain plan has her at 2,033 calories with 56g Fat, 254g Carbs, and 127g Protein. Here are the meal target she set up for herself:

MEAL 1: 455 Calories: 30g Protein (120 Calories), 15g Fat (135 Calories), 50g Carbs (200 Calories)

SNACK: 285 Calories: 10g Protein (40 Calories), 5g Fat (45 Calories), 50g Carbs (200 Calories

MEAL 2: 470 Calories: 35g Protein (140 Calories), 10g Fat (90 Calories), 60g Carbs (240 Calories)

MEAL 3: 600 Calories: 35g Protein (140 Calories), 20g Fat (180 Calories), 70g Carbs (280 Calories)

SNACK: 225 Calories: 20g Protein (80 Calories), 5g Fat (45 Calories), 25g Carbs (100 Calories)

2. FILL YOUR MEALS WITH FOODS YOU ENJOY

What I love most about *Flexible Dieting* is that it's essentially 'structured flexibility.' Your calorie and macro calculations are a guide, but they don't restrict you to any specific food items or rules. I suggest prioritizing nutrient-dense foods at least 80% of the time, and allow 20% to be reserved for discretionary foods. This way you will fill your macro and micronutrient requirements but also find some psychological relief without negative ramifications on your health, quality of life, and goals. When selecting your food sources, it's important to remember that many foods are a combination of macronutrients. If fat loss is the goal, choosing lean proteins for most of your meals (middle list) will help you reach your protein goal easier without consuming excess calories from carbs and fats. I've also provided some cheat sheets for you on proteins, fats, and carbs at the end of this chapter.

Carbs

Pasta, Rice, Bran, Oats, Couscous, Whole Grains, Fruit, Vegetables, Potatoes, Honey, Sugar

Carbs & Protein

Soy, Beans, Peas, Quinoa, Sprouted Grains, Edamame, Tempeh, Non-fat/Low-fat Dairy

Protein

Whey & Casein Protein, Chicken Breast, Turkey Breast, Lean Ground Beef, Bison, Buffalo, Jerky, Tuna, White Fish, Shellfish, Egg Whites

Protein & Fats

Whole Eggs, Salmon, Mackerel, Red Meat, Lamb, Chicken Thigh, Turkey Thigh, Full-fat Dairy, Bacon, Duck, Pork, Cheese, Nuts, Seeds

Fats

Avocado, Olives, Olive Oil, Coconut Oil, Egg Yolks, Flax, Coconut, Mayo, Butter, 90% Dark Chocolate

Pay attention to what foods make you feel good, and what foods don't. Build your personal menu based on the foods that work for you, not whatever is the "super food" of the month.

3. FIND CALORIE-SAVING FOOD SWAPS

Being on a lower calorie diet doesn't mean you can't enjoy the foods you love. There is usually also an alternative to satisfy a craving with a reduced calorie, carb and/or fat option. Low-cal and high-volume food swaps enable you to eat *more* food volume while taking in *fewer* calories. Here are some of my food swaps and kitchen staples for ideas on your next grocery trip:

Full-Fat Dairy → Unsweetened Cashew, Soy and Almond milk, 0% Fat Free Greek Yogurt, Fat Free and Reduced Fat Sour Cream and Cheeses

Ice Cream → Halo Top, Arctic Zero, Fat Free Dryers, Skinny Cow (just don't replace a bowl of ice cream with four bowls or bars of Skinny Cow)

Pasta → Edamame Pasta, Chickpea Pasta, Zucchini Noodles, Sweet Potato Glass Noodles, Rice Noodles, Tofu Noodles, Cauliflower Rice

Chips → Rice Cakes, Air Popped Popcorn, Rice Popped Chips, Quest Protein Chips

Sweets & Treats → Built Bars, Quest Bars, One Bars, Smart Sweets

Bread → Whole Wheat Sandwich Thins, Bagel Thins, English Muffin Thins, Whole Wheat Pita Bread, Low Carb Tortillas, Lettuce Wraps, Jicama Taco Wraps

Bacon, Sausage, Pepperoni → Turkey Bacon, Turkey Pepperoni

Regular Soda → Diet Soda, Sparkling Water, La Croix, Bubbly, Perrier

Fruit Juice → Bai, Vitamin Water Zero, Reduced Sugar Juices (like Trop50)

Condiments → Walden Farms Zero Calorie Sauces and Condiments, Reduced Sugar and Sugar-Free Ketchup and BBQ Sauces, Light Mayo, 0% Greek Yogurt, Light Butter

Sugar → Sugar Substitutes like Stevia, Monk Fruit, Swerve, Splenda, Truvia

Cooking Oils → Fat Free Cooking Sprays

You get the idea. Dare to freestyle with your foods, ingredients, and adjust everything to your taste. Nobody stays on a diet if the food isn't amazing!

HAVE STAPLE FOODS AND EASY RECIPES

A great way I stay on track is having go-to favorite macro-friendly recipes; three to five is good. These serve as staple dishes to make in a pinch, especially in a busy life that is hard pressed for time. I can eat the same thing over and over again. If you get bored easily, pick a few favorite protein sources and build your meals around them, rotating veggies, fruits, and starches. Do yourself a favor and choose foods that are not only healthy, but also convenient and familiar— foods that you and your family really enjoy. This may take some learning and practice, but I promise you'll get the hang of it. I've provided a huge variety of my own **high-protein, low-cal recipes that are** *really* **tasty in Chapter 11**.

 ## MEAL PREP

Meal prep simply means you batch cook recipes and/or prepare ingredients for cooking your meals, or entire meals ahead of time. So once you have your go-to meals and foods, cooking them in bulk will save you precious time during the week. Meal prep can be as simple as making tomorrow's lunch the night before or dedicating a few hours one day of the week to cook meats, starches, and chop vegetables for the week. Store prepped food items in large containers for adding to meals, or even portion full meals in individual containers. How much you meal prep is completely up to you and what works best with your schedule.

Here are the basic questions you can ask yourself as you prepare your meals:

Pick a protein:
- Is there adequate protein? If not, increase portion size.
- Is it a lean protein?
- Is it grilled or poached versus fried? If not, is there a leaner version that can be cooked differently?

Pick at least one vegetable:
- How are the vegetables prepared: raw or cooked?
- If cooked, are they prepared in a healthy manner, such as steamed, grilled or roasted versus breaded or fried?

Pick a healthy, high-fiber starch:
- If grain-based, is it a whole grain or a refined grain?
- Is it prepared in a healthy manner like baked, boiled, or steamed, or does it contain added fat from oil, butter, or cheese?

Pick a healthy fat:
- Is fat included in the preparation of the meal like olive oil, avocado, nuts, seeds?
- Is the amount a healthy portion?

Meal Prep Time Savers:
Grocery stores and deli counters have a variety of grab-and-go packaged foods, cooked meats, chopped veggies and fruit, along with premade salads. Some options may be slightly less healthy than preparing them from scratch and more challenging to track in your app, but these are great time savers! A few of my favorites include:

- Whole, cooked rotisserie chickens
- Pre-hard boiled and peeled eggs
- Individual serving tuna packets
- Pre-chopped fresh vegetables, fruit and packaged salads
- Microwavable rice, potatoes and veggies
- Or: throw a meal together at the salad bar or deli. Beware of creamy dressings, fatty condiments, and fried, oily, fatty meats.

6 PRE-LOG YOUR MEALS

There's no right or wrong way to use a food tracker app, but pre-logging your meals can be helpful in variety of ways:

> Even if you don't meal prep, pre-logging can be handy to track meals and recipes you're planning on making before you prepare them. I always do this so I can change up the ingredients to better suit the macros for the meal I'm making (perhaps a larger serving of protein is needed?). You also have the option to change up other meals in your day to fit around that meal.

> If you meal prep any number of meals for the week, you can pre-log those items in your food tracking app and plan the rest of your meals around them.

> If you're a super planner (I am not...), you can log a full day's worth of food ahead of time so all that is left to do is pack, heat, and eat!

KEEP "SAFE FOODS" ACCESSIBLE

A safe food isn't a "cheat food," but rather a food that you love that doesn't derail your nutrition efforts. One that will satiate and satisfy in the moment, take the edge off a craving, and more importantly, help you reach your goals. For most people, removing every food from the diet that doesn't perfectly fit their macros may work short-term, but eventually, the delightful thought of those "off-limit" foods can lead to a binge-fest! The chocolate fix, for me, is a high-fiber protein bar like Built Bar, or my homemade chocolate chip protein cookies. The sweet flavors satisfy the craving, while the protein and fiber literally fill me up. Yours could be an apple with peanut butter, a banana, or even just a simple square or two of dark chocolate. For others, turkey pepperoni slices, a bag of Quest protein chips, celery with peanut butter, carrots and hummus, or sparkling flavored water will do the trick. My husband, Joel, loves my soft protein pretzels with nacho cheese dip. Just be sure your buffer foods are foods that you CAN stop eating, and **check out my breads, desserts and snack recipes in Chapter 11**. You may find your new favorite "safe food."

 ## HAVE A BACK-UP PLAN

Keeping a supply of healthy frozen meals and go-to restaurant options will enable you to stick to your nutrition goals most of the time.

To make this even easier for you, I've compiled a HUGE list of macro-friendly fast food and restaurant options in Chapter 12.

Meal Timing that Matters

Meal timing, particularly Intermittent Fasting (IF), has become a hot topic in the fitness industry. In fact, Google reports IF as the most popular diet search term in 2019. There are many methods of intermittent fasting, all of which include restricting your food consumption within a window of time. In the hierarchy of importance of weight management, your energy balance (calories consumed versus burned) sits right at the top. Some find restricting food intake to an eight-hour eating window helps them control hunger levels, whereas others may find it makes them ravenously hungry which might result in overeating.

For the average person just trying to lose weight and get healthier, consuming an appropriate amount of calories from a variety of protein, carbs and fat sources is far more important than when the meals are consumed. *Your eating habits should fit into your lifestyle.* If fasting, or any other food timing strategy works for you, then go for it! Just remember that your first priority is whether or not the calories and protein consumed from day to day are in line with your goal.

MAKE YOUR WAY OF EATING WORK FOR YOU!

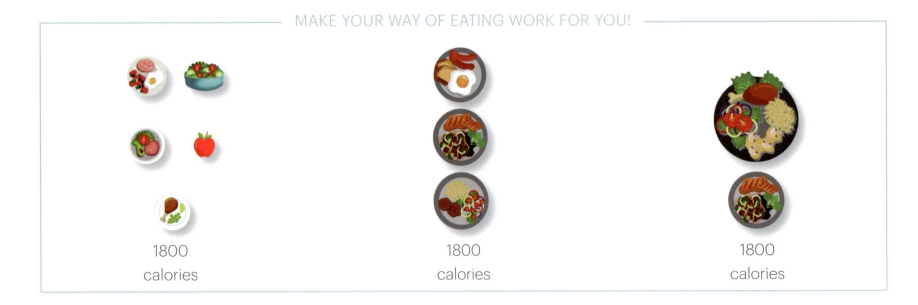

1800 calories   1800 calories   1800 calories

Master Your Macros

Maximizing Muscle Growth with Protein Timing

When it comes to improving your body composition, protein is the super-macronutrient that's going to help you get there (see Chapter 2 for a refresher). For those wanting to *maximize their muscle building potential*, ample evidence supports an advantage with a more strategic approach to protein timing throughout your day.

With each meal, muscle building requires a high-quality protein with a sufficient amount of the branched chain amino acid (BCAA) Leucine to maximize the muscle protein synthesis (MPS). MPS peaks within one and a half hours after consumption and drops to baseline around three hours post meal [92]. A study comparing the rates of MPS over a 12-hour period found that **four equally spaced servings of 20g of whey protein** resulted in higher MPS rates than two servings of 40g of whey protein and eight servings of 10g of whey protein. Essentially, consuming four meals of 20g stimulated MPS more often than two meals of 40g, and 10g was not enough to stimulate MPS at all [93, 91]. A separate study tested 30g of protein spaced between three meals versus 10-15g with breakfast and lunch and about 65g with dinner. Those with an even protein distribution of 30g had 25% greater rates of MPS throughout the day [94]. Thus, equally distributing your daily protein intake between four to five meals around two to three hours apart, including one pre-workout meal can be advantageous when muscle building is a priority [95, 96]. Those who practice intermittent fasting with a short eating window may find that lengthening that window beneficial for optimal protein distribution.

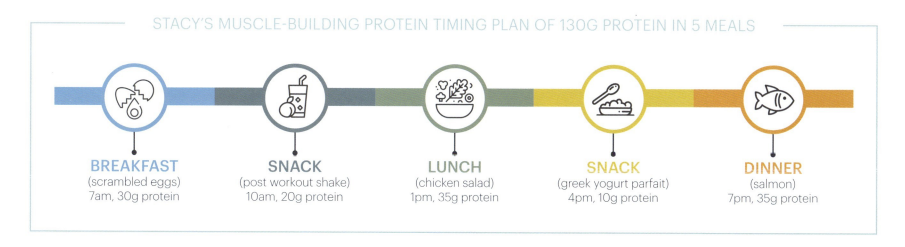

STACY'S MUSCLE-BUILDING PROTEIN TIMING PLAN OF 130G PROTEIN IN 5 MEALS

BREAKFAST (scrambled eggs) 7am, 30g protein

SNACK (post workout shake) 10am, 20g protein

LUNCH (chicken salad) 1pm, 35g protein

SNACK (greek yogurt parfait) 4pm, 10g protein

DINNER (salmon) 7pm, 35g protein

Master Your Macros

How To Read a Nutrition Label

The nutrition label is your *greatest* ally when you're faced with multiple options of similar foods. With so much information on calories, macronutrients, vitamins and minerals it can be a challenge picking one option when you're faced with 20 similar ones at the grocery store. Use this quick scanning strategy to compare between options:

Pay Close Attention: The three features to look at FIRST are number of servings, serving size and calories. If there are eight servings and you eat half of the package, the nutrition facts must be multiplied by four to get an accurate representation of what you consumed.

Minimize: Over-consuming these can add up to a higher risk of high blood pressure and heart disease. US Dietary recommendations: Sodium: 1,500mg max per day. Cholesterol: Eat as little as possible. Foods high in cholesterol like fatty meats and high fat dairy tend to also be high in saturated fats. Saturated fat and added sugars: max 10% daily calories. Trans fats avoid completely.

Maximize: These keep you feeling full, help with fat loss, muscle gain and contribute to improved overall health. US Dietary recommendation of daily fiber is 25g for Women and 38g for Men.

Nutrition Facts

8 Servings per container
Serving size 2/3 cup (55g)

Amount Per Serving
Calories 230

	% Daily Value*
Total Fat 8g	10%
Saturated Fat 1g	5%
Trans Fat 0mg	
Cholesterol 0mg	0%
Sodium 160mg	7%
Total Carbohydrate 37g	13%
Dietary Fiber 4g	14%
Total Sugars 12g	
Includes 10g Added Sugars	20%
Protein 3g	
Vitamin D 2mcg	10%
Calcium 260mg	20%
Iron 8mg	45%
Potassium 235mg	6%

*% **Daily Value** indicates how much one serving of the food item contributes toward a 2,000 daily calorie diet. While your daily calorie goal may differ, the values shown help indicate whether a specific nutrient is high or low. The Academy of Nutrition and Dietetics recommends total fat, saturated fat, cholesterol, and sodium at 5% or less; and fiber, vitamins, and minerals at 20% or more.

Manufacturers are good at creating names, packaging, and claims that make a food appear natural and healthy. The terms Natural, Non-GMO, Cage-Free, Organic or Certified Organic may look encouraging but not all are necessarily meaningful. Compare a few labels of similar products, and you may be surprised what you learn. *Be a critical shopper!*

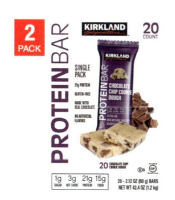

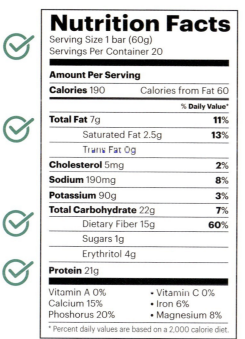

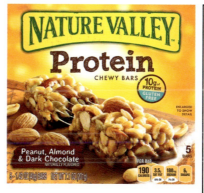

Protein bar provides a larger serving, less saturated fat, more fiber, less sugar, and more protein

Master Your Macros 71

7-Day Meal Plans

Recipes are available in Chapter 12

Jennifer's fat loss meal plan: 1,351 calories/day, 123g Protein, 52g Fat, 97g Carbs:

	SUNDAY	MONDAY	TUESDAY	WEDNESDAY	THURSDAY	FRIDAY	SATURDAY
MEAL 1	Blackberry Ricotta Protein Pancakes, 2 Large Eggs CAL: 376: P: 44g F: 12g C: 24g	Chocolate Peanut Butter Cup Breakfast Bake, 2 Large Eggs CAL: 417: P: 40.5g F: 16g C: 35.5g	Egg & Bacon Breakfast Quesadilla, 1 Peach CAL: 377: P: 32g F: 16g C: 39g	Blackberry Ricotta Protein Pancakes, 2 Large Eggs CAL: 376: P: 44g F: 12g C: 24g	Chocolate Peanut Butter Cup Breakfast Bake, 2 Large Eggs CAL: 417: P: 40.5g F: 16g C: 35.5g	Egg & Bacon Breakfast Quesadilla, 1 Peach CAL: 377: P: 32g F: 16g C: 39g	Blackberry Ricotta Protein Pancakes, 2 Large Eggs CAL: 376: P: 44g F: 12g C: 24g
MEAL 2	Beef Nacho Salad, 1 Orange CAL: 400: P: 36.5g F:12g C: 31.5g	Greek Meatball Wrap w/ Tzatziki Yogurt Sauce, 50g Avocado CAL: 440: P: 40g F: 18g C: 37g	Turkey Sloppy (Thin) Joes, Side Salad w/ Vinaigrette CAL: 413: P: 38g F: 14g C: 40g	Beef Nacho Salad, 1 Orange CAL: 400: P: 36.5g F:12g C: 31.5g	Greek Meatball Wrap w/ Tzatziki Yogurt Sauce, 50g Avocado CAL: 440: P: 40g F: 18g C: 37g	Turkey Sloppy (Thin) Joes, Side Salad w/ Vinaigrette CAL: 413: P: 38g F: 14g C: 40g	Beef Nacho Salad, 1 Orange CAL: 400: P: 36.5g F:12g C: 31.5g
MEAL 3	Turkey Bacon Cheeseburger Flatbread, 1C Roast Veg CAL: 440: P: 47g F: 16g C: 34.5g	Cheesy Beef & Spinach Lasagna Cups (2), Broccolini w/ Lemon & Oil CAL: 430: P: 38g F: 15g C: 41g	Chicken Bacon Ranch Street Tacos (2), 1.5C Steamed Brussels CAL: 422: P: 51g F: 13g C: 44g	Turkey Bacon Cheeseburger Flatbread, 1C Roast Veg CAL: 440: P: 47g F: 16g C: 34.5g	Cheesy Beef & Spinach Lasagna Cups (2), Broccolini w/ Lemon & Oil CAL: 430: P: 38g F: 15g C: 41g	Chicken Bacon Ranch Street Tacos (2), 1.5C Steamed Brussels CAL: 422: P: 51g F: 13g C: 44g	Turkey Bacon Cheeseburger Flatbread, 1C Roast Veg CAL: 440: P: 47g F: 16g C: 34.5g
SNACK	Double Chocolate Protein Donut CAL: 110 P: 13g F: 1g C: 12g	Chocolate Chip Protein Cookies CAL: 81: P: 7.5g F: 2.5g C: 8g	Chocolate Peanut Butter Protein Egg CAL: 148: P: 13 F: 7.5 C: 16	Double Chocolate Protein Donut CAL: 110: P: 13g F: 1g C: 12g	Chocolate Chip Protein Cookies CAL: 81: P: 7.5g F: 2.5g C: 8g	Chocolate Peanut Butter Protein Egg CAL: 148: P: 13 F: 7.5 C: 16	Double Chocolate Protein Donut CAL: 110: P: 13g F: 1g C: 12g
DAILY TOTAL	CAL: 1,326 P: 140.5g, F: 41g, C: 102g	CAL: 1,368 P: 126g, F: 51.5g, C: 121.5g	CAL: 1,360 P: 134g, F: 50.5g, C: 129g	CAL: 1,326 P: 140.5g, F: 41g, C: 102g	CAL: 1,368 P: 126g, F: 51.5g, C: 121.5g	CAL: 1,360 P: 134g, F: 50.5g, C: 129g	CAL: 1,326 P: 140.5g, F: 41g, C: 102g

Master Your Macros

Stacy's muscle gain meal plan: 2,033 calories/day, 127g Protein, 56g Fat, 254g Carbs:

	SUNDAY	MONDAY	TUESDAY	WEDNESDAY	THURSDAY	FRIDAY	SATURDAY
MEAL 1	Cinnamon Roll Protein French Toast CAL: 410: P: 38g, F: 8g, C: 44g	Breakfast Egg Muffins (4), Wheat Toast (2), 2 tbsp Jam CAL: 463: P: 33 F: 12, C: 57	Almond Joy Overnight Oats, Fruit Salad CAL: 524: P: 43g F: 14, C: 69g	Cinnamon Roll Protein French Toast CAL: 410: P: 38g, F: 8g, C: 44g	Breakfast Egg Muffins (4), Wheat Toast (2), 2 tbsp Jam CAL: 463: P: 33, F: 12, C: 57	Almond Joy Overnight Oats, Fruit Salad CAL: 524: P:43g, F: 14, C: 69g	Cinnamon Roll Protein French Toast CAL: 410: P: 38g, F: 8g, C: 44g
SNACK	Banana Chocolate Chip Protein Bread (2), Chai Tea CAL: 388: P: 17g, F: 8g, C: 61g	Spicy Avocado Protein Toast, 1 Banana CAL: 255: P: 11g, F: 7g, C: 48g	Soft Protein Pretzel with Nacho Cheese Dip, 1 Apple CAL: 308: P: 20g, F: 4g, C: 51g	Banana Chocolate Chip Protein Bread (2), Chai Tea CAL: 388: P: 17g, F: 8g, C: 61g	Spicy Avocado Protein Toast, 1 Banana CAL: 255: P: 11g, F: 7g, C: 48g	Soft Protein Pretzel with Nacho Cheese Dip, 1 Apple CAL: 308: P: 20g, F: 4g, C: 51g	Banana Chocolate Chip Protein Bread (2), Chai Tea CAL: 388: P: 17g, F: 8g, C: 61g
MEAL 2	Spicy Beef Mac & Cheese, Side Salad, Small Apple CAL: 497: P: 40g, F: 14g, C: 57g	Apple Walnut Tuna Salad Wrap, 1C Baby Carrots, Vanilla Yogurt CAL: 524, P: 36g, F: 14g, C: 64g	Egg Salad Slimwich, Baked Tortilla Chips & Salsa CAL: 451: P: 34g, F: 14g, C: 56g	Spicy Beef Mac & Cheese, Side Salad, Small Apple CAL: 497: P: 40g, F: 14g, C: 57g	Apple Walnut Tuna Salad Wrap, 1C Baby Carrots, Vanilla Yogurt CAL: 524, P: 36g, F: 14g, C: 64g	Egg Salad Slimwich, Baked Tortilla Chips & Salsa CAL: 451, P: 34g, F: 14g, C: 56g	Spicy Beef Mac & Cheese, Side Salad, Small Apple CAL: 497: P: 40g, F: 14g, C: 57g
MEAL 3	Turkey Enchiladas, 1/2C Rice, 1C Roasted Veg CAL: 587: P: 34g, F: 19g, C: 80g	Blackbean Quesadilla Burger, 2C Roasted Veg CAL: 552: P: 35g, F: 25g, C: 66g	Pepperoni Protein Pizza, Large Salad, 6oz. Glass of Wine CAL: 574: P: 35g, F:19g, C: 29g	Turkey Enchiladas, 1/2C Rice, 1C Roasted Veg CAL: 587: P: 34g, F: 19g, C: 80g	Blackbean Quesadilla Burger, 2C Roasted Veg CAL: 552: P: 35g F: 25g, C: 66g	Pepperoni Protein Pizza, Large Salad, 6oz. Glass of Wine CAL: 574: P: 35g, F:19g, C: 29g	Turkey Enchiladas, 1/2C Rice, 1C Roasted Veg CAL: 587: P: 34g, F: 19g, C: 80g
SNACK	Chocolate Peanut Butter Protein Egg CAL: 148, P: 13, F: 7.5, C: 16	Confetti Cake Protein Dip (2), 1/2 Apple CAL: 220: P 13g, F: 6g, C: 31g	Chocolate Chip Protein Cookie Dough CAL: 168: P: 18g, F: 4g, C: 23g	Chocolate Peanut Butter Protein Egg CAL: 148: P: 13, F: 7.5, C: 16	Confetti Cake Protein Dip (2), 1/2 Apple CAL: 220, P 13g, F: 6g, C: 31g	Chocolate Chip Protein Cookie Dough CAL: 168: P: 18g, F: 4g, C: 23g	Chocolate Peanut Butter Protein Egg CAL: 148: P: 13, F: 7.5, C: 16
DAILY TOTAL	CAL: 2,030 P: 142g, F: 56g, C: 258g	CAL: 2,014 P: 128g, F: 64g, C: 266g	CAL: 2,025 P: 150g, F: 55g, C: 228g	CAL: 2,030 P: 142g, F: 56g, C: 258g	CAL: 2,014 P: 128g, F: 64g, C: 266g	CAL: 2,025 P: 150g, F: 55g, C: 228g	CAL: 2,030 P: 142g, F: 56g, C: 258g

Master Your Macros

Protein Cheat Sheet

A few animal-based protein sources to use in your meal plan.

CHICKEN BREAST
4 OZ. (SKINLESS)

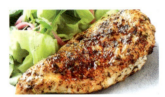

160 CALORIES
30G PROTEIN

GROUND BEEF
4 OZ. (93% LEAN)

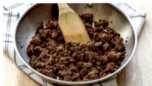

220 CALORIES
25G PROTEIN

TURKEY BREAST
4 OZ. (99% LEAN)

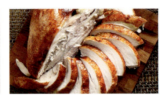

160 CALORIES
30G PROTEIN

ALBACORE TUNA
4 OZ. (IN WATER)

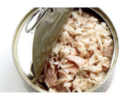

120 CALORIES
26G PROTEIN

LIQUID EGG WHITES
1 CUP

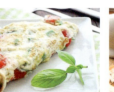

120 CALORIES
28G PROTEIN

PORK TENDERLOIN
4 OZ.

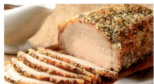

167 CALORIES
29G PROTEIN

VENISON
4 OZ.

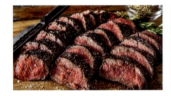

178 CALORIES
25G PROTEIN

LAMB
4 OZ.

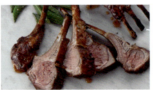

320 CALORIES
19G PROTEIN

COD
4 OZ.

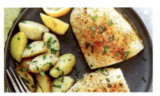

119 CALORIES
26G PROTEIN

SHRIMP
4 OZ.

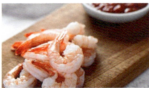

107 CALORIES
24G PROTEIN

WILD SALMON
4 OZ.

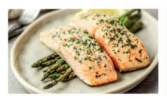

233 CALORIES
29G PROTEIN

TILAPIA
4 OZ.

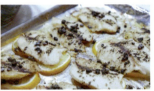

145 CALORIES
30G PROTEIN

0% GREEK YOGURT
6 OZ.

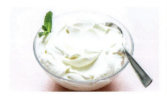

90 CALORIES
18G PROTEIN

NON-FAT COTTAGE CHEESE
6 OZ.

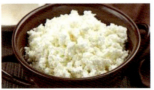

120 CALORIES
21G PROTEIN

BEEF/TURKEY JERKY
1 OZ.

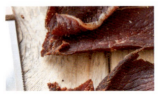

90 CALORIES
10G PROTEIN

WHEY PROTEIN
1 SCOOP

120 CALORIES
24G PROTEIN

WHEY PROTEIN BAR
1 SERVING

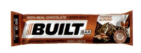

110-200 CALORIES
15-21G PROTEIN

CASEIN PROTEIN
1 SCOOP

120 CALORIES
24G PROTEIN

Master Your Macros

Vegan Protein Cheat Sheet

A few plant-based protein sources to use in your meal plan. *Indicates a complete protein source.

*QUINOA
1/2 CUP

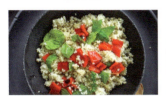

110 CALORIES
4G PROTEIN

*TOFU
4 OZ.

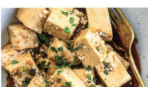

95 CALORIES
10G PROTEIN

*TVP (TEXTURED VEGETABLE PROTEIN)
1/2 CUP

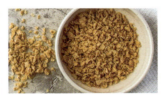

180 CALORIES
26G PROTEIN

*TEMPEH
4 OZ.

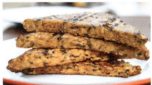

220 CALORIES
21G PROTEIN

SEITAN (VITAL WHEAT GLUTEN)
4 OZ.

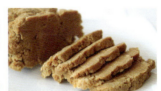

104 CALORIES
21G PROTEIN

NUTRITIONAL YEAST
1/2 CUP

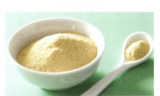

120 CALORIES
16G PROTEIN

SPROUTED WHOLE GRAIN BREAD 2 SLICES

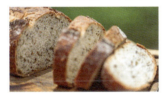

160 CALORIES
8G PROTEIN

*EDAMAME
1/2 CUP

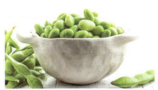

127 CALORIES
11G PROTEIN

CHICKPEAS
1/2 CUP

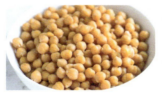

143 CALORIES
6G PROTEIN

BLACK BEANS
1/2 CUP

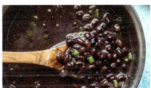

114 CALORIES
7.5G PROTEIN

LENTILS
1/2 CUP

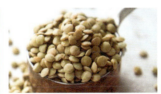

120 CALORIES
9G PROTEIN

SUNFLOWER SEEDS
1/2 CUP

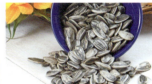

320 CALORIES
14G PROTEIN

HEMP SEEDS
1/2 CUP

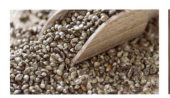

480 CALORIES
26G PROTEIN

POWDERED PEANUT BUTTER 1/2 CUP

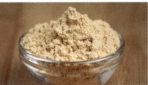

180 CALORIES
20G PROTEIN

PEANUT BUTTER
2 TBSP

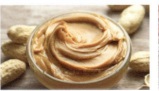

188 CALORIES
8G PROTEIN

ALMONDS
1/2 CUP

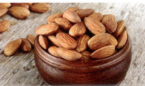

243 CALORIES
9G PROTEIN

*RICE & PEA PROTEIN
1 SCOOP

180 CALORIES
20G PROTEIN

*VEGAN PROTEIN BAR
1 SERVING

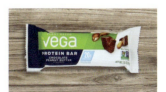

200-300 CALORIES
15-20G PROTEIN

Fat Cheat Sheet

A few fat sources high in Omega 3 and 6 to use in your meal plan.

WILD SALMON
4 OZ.
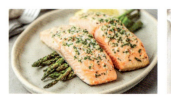
233 CALORIES
13G FAT

HERRING
4 OZ.
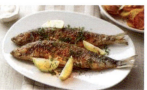
246 CALORIES
14G FAT

MACKEREL
4 OZ.
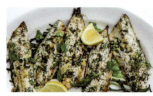
293 CALORIES
20G FAT

LARGE EGGS
4 WHOLE
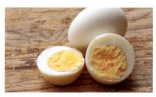
280 CALORIES
16G FAT

AVOCADO
1/2 LARGE
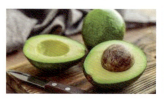
161 CALORIES
15G FAT

OLIVES
3 OZ.
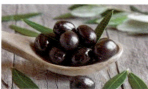
100 CALORIES
9G FAT

WALNUTS
1 OZ.
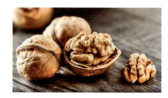
150 CALORIES
10G FAT

ALMOND BUTTER
2 TBSP
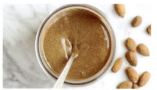
203 CALORIES
19G FAT

PECANS
1 OZ.
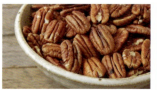
190 CALORIES
20G FAT

MACADAMIA NUTS
1 OZ.
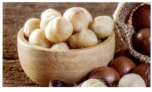
220 CALORIES
22G FAT

CHIA SEEDS
2 TBSP
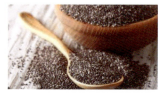
130 CALORIES
7G FAT

SUNFLOWER SEEDS
2 TBSP
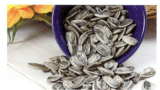
169 CALORIES
16G FAT

OYSTERS
4 OZ.
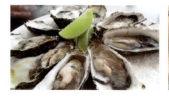
121 CALORIES
5G FAT

FLAXSEED
2 TBSP (WHOLE)
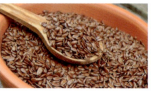
112 CALORIES
9G FAT

COCONUT OIL
1 TBSP
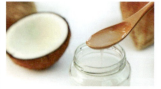
120 CALORIES
14G FAT

FLAXSEED OIL
1 TBSP
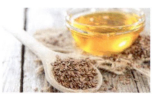
120 CALORIES
14G FAT

OLIVE OIL
1 TBSP
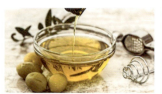
120 CALORIES
14G FAT

MCT OIL
1 TBSP
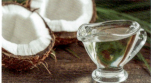
130 CALORIES
14G FAT

Carb Cheat Sheet

A few high-fiber options to use in your meal plan.

OATMEAL 1/2 CUP	**BROWN RICE** 1/2 CUP	**SWEET POTATO** MEDIUM 5"	**BRAN CEREAL** 1/2 CUP	**NAVY BEANS** 1/2 CUP	**BULGUR** 1/2 CUP
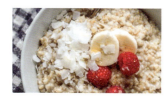	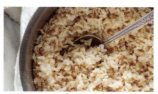	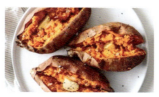	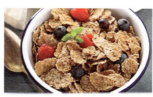	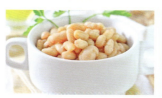	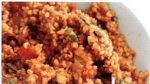
150 CALORIES 27G CARBS/ 4G FIBER	150 CALORIES 34G CARBS/ 2G FIBER	112 CALORIES 26G CARBS/ 4G FIBER	90 CALORIES 20G CARBS/ 13G FIBER	127 CALORIES 24G CARBS/ 9.5G FIBER	50 CALORIES 15G CARBS/ 4G FIBER
WHOLE WHEAT PASTA 1/2 CUP	**PUMPKIN** 5 OZ.	**KIDNEY BEANS** 1/2 CUP	**LENTILS** 1/2 CUP	**ARTICHOKE** 1 WHOLE	**BANANA** MEDIUM 7"
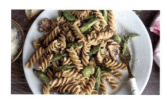	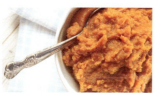	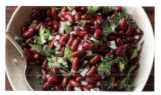	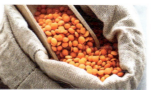	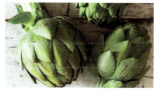	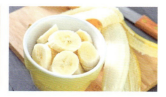
87 CALORIES 19G CARBS/ 3G FIBER	46 CALORIES 10G CARBS/ 4G FIBER	90 CALORIES 19G CARBS/ 8G FIBER	115 CALORIES 20G CARBS /7.8G FIBER	76 CALORIES 17G CARBS/ 8.5G FIBER	105 CALORIES 27G CARBS/ 3G FIBER
GALA APPLE MEDIUM	**ORANGE** MEDIUM	**BLACKBERRIES** 1/2 CUP	**RASPBERRIES** 1/2 CUP	**BROCCOLI** 1 CUP	**CARROTS** 1 CUP
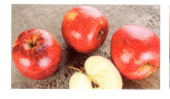	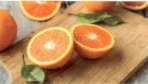	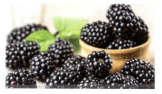	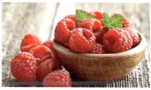	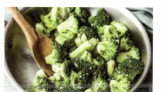	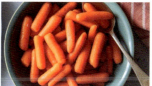
95 CALORIES 25G CARBS/ 4G FIBER	62 CALORIES 15G CARBS/ 3G FIBER	35 CALORIES 9G CARBS/ 3G FIBER	35 CALORIES 8G CARBS/ 4G FIBER	20 CALORIES 4G CARBS/ 2G FIBER	52 CALORIES 12G CARBS/ 4G FIBER

Master Your Macros

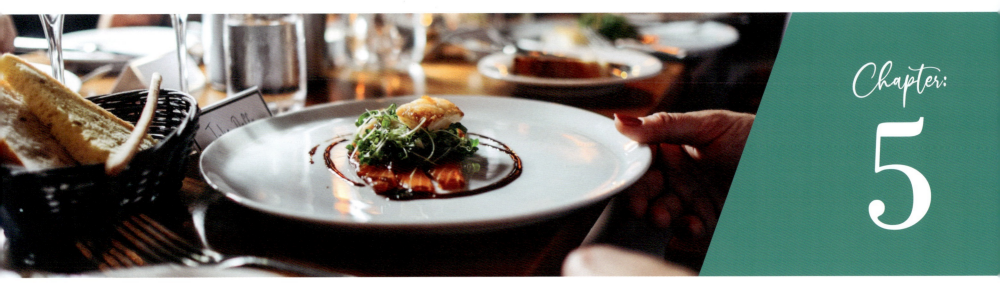

Factor In Your Fun

Think about how awesome it will be to eat out, travel, and indulge in treats you love and not lose all of your gains! How about coming back from a vacation lighter than you started? Yes! This is the reality I discovered when I embraced *Flexible Dieting*. This is by far the best approach to stay on track and see results, regardless of where you are.

The recommendations I've put together in this chapter will empower you to make choices that support your goals when dining out or away from home. Keep in mind it is totally ok to head out to your favorite restaurant, or somewhere new and exciting and eat a meal that is not tracked and counted. We're not here to be macro-tracking robots if we also can't live a life we enjoy!

The Dish on Dining Out

Dining out and traveling present their own challenges when trying to eat healthy. But the good news is all it takes is a little planning, and healthy choices are possible in any situation. Remember that change of any kind takes repetition, practice, and perseverance. Many restaurants, especially chains and fast food spots, publish their menu with nutrition information online. All that's left for you to do is plan for what you want and work the rest of your day around it.

Even better, I've already done a lot of the research for you! Check out my hand-picked macro-friendly meals from over 50 fast food and restaurant chains in Chapter 12.

STEP 1
Find Your Meal **Ahead of Time**

see what's on the menu | look up the nutrition info

STEP 2
Plan to Order **What You Want**

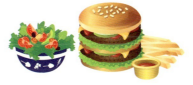

(just be reasonable)

STEP 3
Make Your **Other Meals Fit**

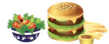

If your daily goal is 1800 cals & dinner is 1000 cals...

Maybe use... **300 Calories** for breakfast & **500 Calories** for lunch?

STEP 4
You Won't Be Perfect...**That's Okay!**

Be as accurate as you can, but don't stress if you go over a little.

Pre-planning works well when the information is available. More often than not, I have found that planning ahead isn't an option. Here are a few strategies I use that will help you stay on track at any restaurant.

>> Avoid Arriving Ravenous

Letting yourself get too hungry before dining out increases chances of overeating the bread basket or other appetizers, along with picking a meal that doesn't fit your goals. A small high-protein snack an hour before dinner will curve your appetite and help you make better decisions when you arrive.

>> Set Checks & Balances

Appetizers, alcohol, oversized meals and desserts provide many opportunities to go overboard. Skip on the foods you're not crazy about, eat normal portion sizes, and share something more indulgent with the rest of the table.

>> Prioritize Protein & Veggies

Prioritizing lean protein appetizers and meals will help you meet your daily target and feel more satisfied on fewer calories. Vegetables tend to be low-calorie, but they still fill you up with extra food volume, fiber, vitamins and minerals.

>> Choose Between Carbs or Fat

Foods that are high in carbs and fats are usually the most calorie-dense. Pizza, creamy pasta and fried foods are common examples. Choose a meal either higher in carbs or fats, but not both.

>> Beware of Hidden Calories, Sides, and Sauces

Request limited oil or butter be used when cooking your meal. Ask for salad dressings and sauces/dips to be served on the side. Opt for steamed veggies or a house salad in place of sides like fries, garlic bread, or mashed potatoes. Watch portion sizes of fats like nuts, cheese, and avocado. They'll add a lot of calories to your meal quickly.

>> Understand the Menu

Steamed, blackened, poached, broiled, baked, grilled, and roasted mean the meal was cooked with little to no oils or creams. Au gratin, basted, braised, buttered, creamed, scalloped, fried/crispy, cheese/butter cream sauce, gravy, pan fried, pan roasted, and sautéed pack on calories and fat with added oils, cheese, and creams used during the cooking process.

Best Restaurant Food Options

Bar Food

Avoid foods that are fried such as onion rings, French fries, fried chicken wings, or fried spring rolls. Steer clear of cheese and cream-based dishes like jalapeno poppers, loaded nachos and potato skins, spinach and artichoke dip, mozzarella sticks, ranch, blue cheese and Caesar dressings.

- Chicken Tenders
- Chicken Satay and Skewers
- Shrimp Cocktail
- Baked Meatballs
- Hummus and Pita bread
- Lettuce Wraps or Soft Tacos with Chicken or Shrimp and Vegetables
- Grilled Calamari

Mexican

Choose grilled fish or chicken, brown rice, a smaller serving of cheese (or none), black beans over refried beans and corn tortillas over flour. Avoid fried foods like taquitos, empanadas and chimichangas. Opt for salsa and/or a little guacamole over sour cream and cheese.

- Fajitas
- Burrito Bowls
- Soft Shell Tacos
- Grilled fish
- Grilled Chicken
- Mexican Salads

Italian

Opt for whole grain pasta if available or brown rice in your risotto. Choose tomato over cream-based sauces. Look for vegetable-based dishes since Italian can be unbalanced in terms of carb, protein and fat ratio.

- Minestrone Soup
- Grilled or Baked Fish
- Italian Salads, dressing on the side
- Chicken Pasta Primavera
- Bruschetta

Thai

Be aware of cream-based curries which add extra calories and fat. Avoid deep fried entrees such as spring rolls, crispy chicken, salt and pepper squid.

- Tofu
- Chicken
- Vegetable-based Stir Fries
- Pad Thai
- Fresh Spring Rolls
- Soup

Sushi

Avoid anything tempura, fried and crunchy and creamy mayo sauces. "Fancier" rolls, such as rainbow, dynamite or spider are larger and have more ingredients, therefore are higher in calories. Add avocado to only one of your rolls to keep calories under control.

- Edamame
- Sashimi
- Miso soup
- Fresh Tuna, Yellow tail, Shrimp, Salmon
- Veggie rolls

Indian

Avoid fried entrees such as pakoras and samosas. Look out for the words 'paneer', 'ghee' and 'malai', these are all higher calorie options that include cheeses, cream and butter based.

- Lentil-based Dals
- Tandoori Kebabs
- Salads
- Chana Masala
- Aloo Gobi

Pizza

Since nearly all the protein options are higher fat and higher calorie, going strictly veggies reduces calories a ton. Opt for chicken breast, Canadian bacon, or get your protein elsewhere! While cauliflower crust options can be slightly lower in calories, they're also lower in fiber and protein than whole wheat options. Gluten-free crusts are ideal for those with gluten sensitivities.

- Thin, Whole Wheat Crust
- Light Cheese
- Veggie Toppings

Chinese

Many entrées are battered, deep fried, and typically loaded with salt, sugar, and oil. Avoid dishes with thicker and stickier sauces, like General Tso's and sweet and sour, which are higher in sugar and calories. Opt for sauce on the side, garlic sauce, brown over white rice, and dishes with lots of vegetables that are baked, steamed, boiled, or sautéed in a small amount of oil.

- Beef & Broccoli
- Chicken & Broccoli
- Chop Suey
- Steamed Dumplings
- Hot & Sour / Egg Drop Soup
- Egg Foo Young
- Buddha's Delight

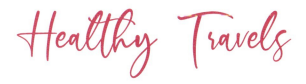
Healthy Travels

When we travel, there are many different problems that may derail us from hitting our macros. Protein is already the hardest to hit for most, but when traveling, you have to be proactive to ensure you're eating enough. Carbs and fat are extremely easy to come by, so be mindful and don't go overboard on them.

My husband, Joel, and I travel a lot! So, if you get one tip out of this chapter, pay close attention to this: *at every meal take in as much protein and fiber as you can!* This will ensure that you are full, will limit cravings and save you from going nuts on all the goodies that will present themselves. This tip solves 80% of your nutrition struggles while traveling!

Eating out will likely make up a majority of your meals, so the dining out tips listed above should be extremely helpful. Although most hotels do not have a kitchen, many will have a small fridge which can provide the opportunity to make small meals in your room. For longer trips, staying in a condo or AirBnB with a kitchen provides the opportunity to grocery shop and cook as many meals as you would at home. **I also find it handy to pack a supply of my favorite portable snacks so I'm not limited to gas station snacks, airport food, and fast food restaurants along the way.**

Protein Bars ie. Built Bar, Quest, One
Protein Chips ie. Quest, IWON Organics
Beef and Turkey Jerky
Hard Boiled Eggs
Tuna Packets
Babybel and String Cheese
Veggies ie. baby carrots, celery, cucumber, zucchini
Fruit ie. apples, oranges, bananas, berries, clementine's
Applesauce packets
Hummus Cups
Oatmeal Cups
Rice Cakes
Air Popped Popcorn
Dry Cereal ie. Protein Cheerios, Kashi Go-Lean, Bran, Fiber One
Almond & Peanut Butter Packets
Nuts and Seeds
Roasted Seaweed Snacks
Smart Sweets

The Truth about Alcohol

Alcohol provides 7.1 calories per gram (ouch!), which is double that of protein and carbs and slightly below fat. Unlike protein, carbs, and fat, alcohol is non-essential for bodily functions— in fact, it's technically a toxin— so the body has no storage capacity for it. This means that after ingestion, alcohol must be metabolized before any food consumed with it is utilized. But there are some caveats.

You may know that alcoholic drinks tend to be high in un-satiating calories, but when you combine that with those intra and post-drinking food binges, caloric intake can go through the roof. For example, I love wine, but I know that two standard glasses is about 300 calories. If I were to add an appetizer, slice of lasagna, roasted veggies, two pieces of garlic bread and a heaping scoop of ice cream, my meal has easily exceeded 1,300 calories! Those 1,000+ food calories will not be used as fuel by my body until it has eliminated the wine first. This is why those trying to lose fat may struggle if they consume alcohol.

I have good news! As long as protein intake is met and calories are accounted for, alcohol consumed in *moderation* is not associated with weight gain, nor will it interfere with muscle building [97]. Interestingly, individuals who consume alcohol in moderate amounts have a reduced risk of becoming overweight, or developing coronary heart disease and type 2 diabetes than abstainers and heavy drinkers [97, 98].

When your body composition goal is top priority, I suggest limiting alcohol to two to three drinks per week. Alcohol straight, on the rocks or with a low-calorie /zero-calorie mixer like soda water, diet soda, light cranberry juice, lemon or lime juice will reduce overall calorie intake.

Alcohol Cheat Sheet

TYPES OF ALCOHOL

Drink	Serving	Calories	ABV
Champagne	5 fl oz	96	12.5%
Vodka	1.5 fl oz	96	40%
Gin	1.5 fl oz	96	40%
Rum	1.5 fl oz	97	40%
Tequila	1.5 fl oz	104	40%
Scotch	1.5 fl oz	105	40%
Whiskey	1.5 fl oz	105	40%
Cinnamon Whiskey	1.5 fl oz	108	33%
Light Beer	12 oz (1 can)	110	4.2%
Brandy	1.5 fl oz	115	40%
White Wine	5 fl oz	121	12.5%
Red Wine	5 fl oz	125	14%
Coffee Liqueur	1.5 fl oz	137	20%
Beer	12 oz (1 can)	145	5%
Hard Cider	12 oz	150	5%

COMMON COCKTAILS

Cocktail	Serving	Calories
Vodka Soda	8 fl oz	96
Gin & Tonic	8 fl oz	161
Mojito	3.5 fl oz	169
Rum & Coke	8 fl oz	173
Sangria	5 fl oz	175
Manhattan	3.5 fl oz	200
Cosmopolitan	3.5 fl oz	211
Martini	3.5 fl oz	215
Daquiri	3.5 fl oz	229
Whiskey Sour	3.5 fl oz	240
Pina Colada	3.5 fl oz	242
Magarita	3.5 fl oz	254

Master Your Macros

When to Treat Yourself

Absence makes the heart grow fonder, so completely eliminating the foods you enjoy will only increase your desire for them. So, please don't ask me to give up peanut butter or chocolate! Research shows if a little room isn't left for the foods you love, the more likely you are to eventually binge, overeat, or quit your diet all together [100, 101].

Flexible approaches to nutrition, as I've been outlining in this guide, allow for occasional divergence from plans. Yes, you can enjoy an occasional treat on your diet. Here's why: Flexible Dieting has been linked to lower calorie intakes, and therefore, greater weight loss [102]! Successful dieters understand that foods aren't 'good' or 'bad," some are just more nutrient-dense and do a better job supporting your health and goals than others. When you enjoy nutritious foods a *majority of the time*, an occasional treat or "cheat meal" will offer a much needed psychological break along with a decrease in food cravings [92]. The most important thing I want to emphasize is not to allow the occasional treat, cheat, or day-off derail you or make you feel bad. Adherence to your nutrition plan long-term is the key to getting results and keeping them!

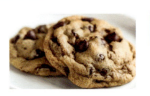

Emotion

"This cookie is a 'junk food' and eating it will make me fat."

Science

It's 200 enjoyable calories with minimal nutrients.

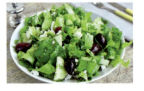

"Eating this salad is healthy and will make me thin."

Salads don't cause weight loss, an overall calorie deficit does.

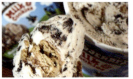

"I have been bad and ruined all my progress; I might as well eat this whole tub of ice cream."

You consumed 300 unplanned calories, then another 1,000 out of guilt. The latter is the part that ruined your calorie deficit.

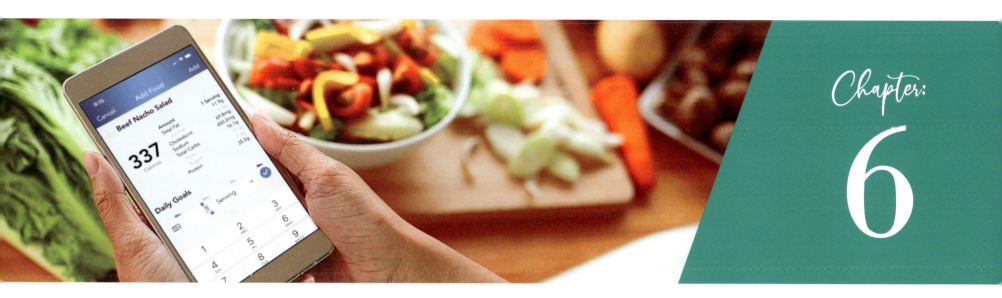

Chapter: 6

Lets Get Tracking

Tracking is not as difficult or complicated as many think, especially in the digital age. Smartphone apps, like *Lose It!*, can do most of the work for you. Researchers have concluded that self-monitoring food intake through tracking is the number one predictor of fat-loss. And the studies show that those who diligently use smartphone apps lose nearly double the body fat and keep it off longer [103,104]!

The "Spark" that Gets Things Going

Losing fat and building muscle typically requires you to adopt and maintain a combination of new behaviors. Eat better. Move more. Lift. Find ways to make unhealthy environments healthy. Change your social environment so it supports your healthy decisions. Reframe how you react in a high-calorie social setting.

Even though a lot of this can make you groan inside, in my experience, food tracking is a straightforward behavior that improves more complex behaviors as you navigate your journey. It's the first step–or spark–that gets things going.

Tracking works for newbies and experienced physique athletes alike. Newbies need to do it, at least for a while, because in many cases, it's a very eye-opening experience. Whereas advanced physique athletes know when it's time to dial things in and get strict; the numbers set them straight. When you track, you see first-hand how each food you eat impacts your daily calorie and macro targets. This data can tell you where to make changes and what foods fit into your macros like a glove.

First Things First

There are many apps out there, so use one you enjoy and are comfortable with. This chapter will guide you through the *Lose It!* app. Basic features are always free. Premium features come with a small annual fee or lifetime membership flat rate.

My gift to you is a 7-day *Lose It!* premium trial, so why not give it a try at http://fbuy.me/v/breannefreeman

"Master Your Macros" is an independent publication and has not been authorized, sponsored, or otherwise approved by FitNow, Inc., d/b/a *Lose It!*.

Get Your App Set Up to Track

Set up the "About You" section with the personal data and the activity factor you used to calculate your calories and macros in Chapter 3. The number displayed is what the app calculated as your Total Daily Energy Expenditure (TDEE). This number should be within 100 calories of your calculations in Chapter 3. Remember, there are different BMR and TDEE mathematical models, and each is based on averages of large populations. Neither is "more accurate" because calories in and out isn't an exact science.

Set the Rate in "**My Calorie Budget**" to match your weekly weight loss goal. The final calorie goal should be close to your calculations in Chapter 3. You can manually adjust the *Lose It!* calculations (increase or decrease calories) by tapping the "**Adjust Budget...**"

If your primary goal is weight maintenance or muscle gain, keep your weight loss rate at 0 pounds per week and "**Adjust Budget...**" to increase daily calories for your goal.

Customize Your Goals

The free version of *Lose It!* provides insights on the protein, carbs, and fat you have consumed daily. Premium members can track various custom goals, all of which are managed under the "Goals" tab. At a minimum, protein, carbohydrates, and fat goals can be set in grams per day based on your calculations from Chapter 3. Creating custom goals is also a great opportunity to track U.S. dietary guidelines for fiber (25g for women, 38g for men per day), saturated fat and sugar do not exceed 10% daily calories, and sodium not to exceed 2,300mg per day [104]. Other helpful goals include water intake, steps, body fat %, even sleep. Over time, and patterns on each goal will emerge.

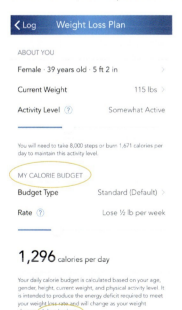
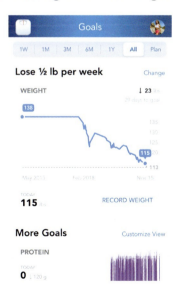

Download *Lose It!* http://fbuy.me/v/breannefreeman

What's on Your Screen

Once you have set up your calories, macros, and meal settings in your *Lose It!* app, you're ready to start tracking. Here's a little walkthrough of your home screen and what each icon means.

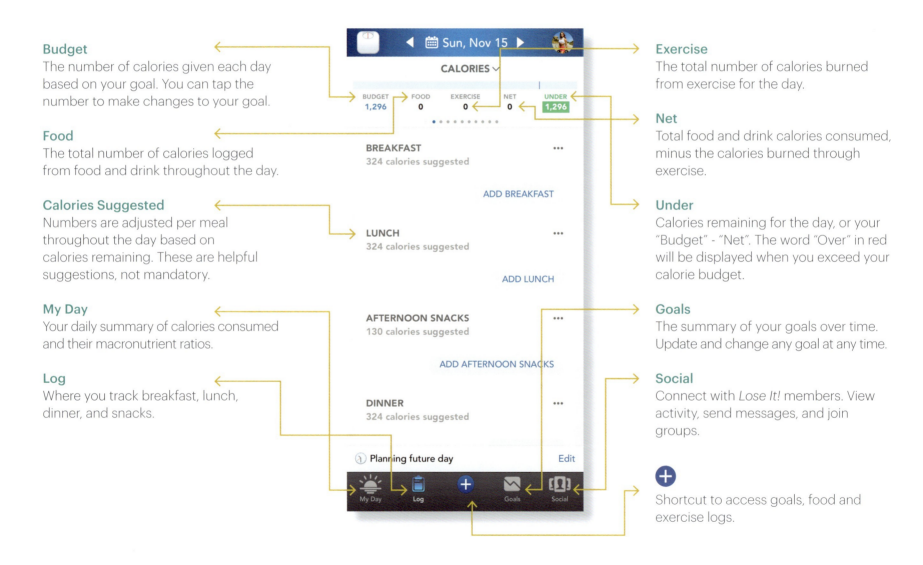

Budget
The number of calories given each day based on your goal. You can tap the number to make changes to your goal.

Food
The total number of calories logged from food and drink throughout the day.

Calories Suggested
Numbers are adjusted per meal throughout the day based on calories remaining. These are helpful suggestions, not mandatory.

My Day
Your daily summary of calories consumed and their macronutrient ratios.

Log
Where you track breakfast, lunch, dinner, and snacks.

Exercise
The total number of calories burned from exercise for the day.

Net
Total food and drink calories consumed, minus the calories burned through exercise.

Under
Calories remaining for the day, or your "Budget" - "Net". The word "Over" in red will be displayed when you exceed your calorie budget.

Goals
The summary of your goals over time. Update and change any goal at any time.

Social
Connect with *Lose It!* members. View activity, send messages, and join groups.

+
Shortcut to access goals, food and exercise logs.

Download *Lose It!* http://fbuy.me/v/breannefreeman

Master Your Macros

Enter Foods into Your Log

Don't think you can't track it all. If you're eating it, chances are *Lose It!* has it with a database of over 33 million foods! Since you'll be entering food several times a day, *Lose It!* makes this task fast and easy with multiple ways of doing it:

Search, My Foods, Meals, Brands

Type in keywords to find your previously entered foods, entire meals, food brands, or restaurant meals (Campbells, Quest, Wendy's, Cheesecake Factory, etc.). Adjust for the correct serving size and add it to your log. Remember when creating a custom entry, the more nutrition values you enter, the better your insights will be.

Smart Camera Functionality

Log just about any food item in a snap! Tap the … symbol on the meal or snack you want to log. Select "Scan Barcode, Nutrition or Food." Using your phone's camera, hover over the barcode, nutrition label, or food item and the app will do the work for you! Review your selection for accuracy, confirm serving size, and add to your log.

Verified Foods

Foods with the green checkmark have been verified by the *Lose It!* Food Database Team and believed to be accurate with complete nutritional data. Unverified foods have been added by *Lose It!* members, like you and me. While unverified foods can be correct and complete, I have found many just include a calorie count. If your food doesn't have a label and the entry seems off, you can double-check with http://nutritiondata.self.com/.

Recipes

Create and save your database of recipes right in the app. Add each individual ingredient, specify the number of servings, and the app calculates the calories and macros of each serving for you (woo-hoo!). All that's left to do is add the recipe serving(s) to your log. When you make that recipe again, all the hard work is done. You can even share your recipes with other *Lose It!* users!

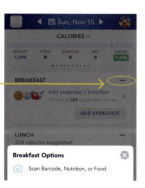
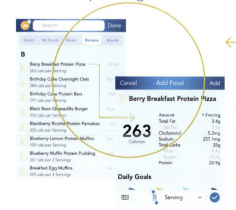

Download *Lose It!* http://fbuy.me/v/breannefreeman

How to Track Meals Out

If nutrition facts aren't available at the restaurant you're dining at (check the *Lose It!* app and the restaurant website), you'll need to add each ingredient of your meal to your *Lose It!* log. The menu should list all the ingredients; if not, ask your server. Don't forget about things like oils and sauces, as these are often not as visible in the dish but tend to be more calorie-dense. Log in some extra olive oil if the meal seems particularly oily. Spices and sodium don't contain calories, so you don't need to worry about them for weight gain or weight loss. Here are some visual guidelines that may help.

A TEASPOON
4 grams
A serving of oil =
1 DICE

A TABLESPOON
14 grams
A condiment serving =
BOTTLE CAP / POKER CHIP

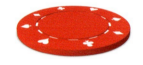

A QUARTER CUP
85 grams
A serving of nuts =
1 LARGE EGG

A HALF CUP
170 grams
A serving of cooked rice =
HOCKEY PUCK / TENNIS BALL

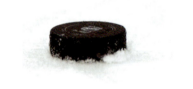

ONE CUP
340 grams
A serving of fruits /
vegetables = BASEBALL

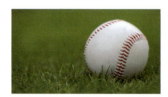

THREE OUNCES
85 grams
A small meat serving =
DECK OF CARDS

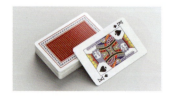

FOUR - FIVE OUNCES
113-142 grams
A medium meat serving =
REGULAR SMARTPHONE

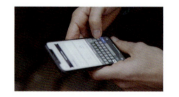

EIGHT - NINE OUNCES
227-255 grams
Restaurant burgers & fish =
LARGE SMARTPHONE

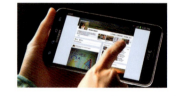

The Little Things Add Up

Some find success in logging all their food ahead of time while others log as they go. There is no right or wrong way, so do what works best for you and keep these tips in mind:

Weigh & Measure
Weighing food will provide the most accuracy, more so than measuring cups and spoons. I've provided some easy food scale instructions at the end of this chapter to get you started. If you don't have a scale, do your best to be accurate with your measuring tools.

Serving Size Matters
Check the nutrition label for actual serving count and size. What you think is a single-serving package may contain two or more servings, which means you just took in twice the calories or more than you thought.

The Extras Count
Don't forget those little bites and nibbles, cream and sugar, salad dressings, sauces, and oils used to cook your food. Two tablespoons of coffee creamer: 40 calories; a handful of croutons: 100 calories; a tablespoon of sunflower seeds: 50 calories. A smear of almond butter on your apple, a dollop of mayonnaise in your tuna salad—it all adds up.

Liquid Calories Are Sneaky
Be aware of calories in sweetened teas, coffee drinks, lemonade, fruit juices, and vegetable juices. Trendy chia seed drinks and kombucha can have 200+ calories a bottle. Check the nutrition label and account for it in your daily calorie budget.

Success with your nutrition plan is as much about perspective as it is adherence and consistency.

"NOT WORTH TRACKING"

30 cal   30 cal   30 cal

250 cal   250 cal   250 cal

304 cal   50 cal   42 cal

3X30G KETCHUP, 3X30G MAYO, 30G BBQ SAUCE, 30G BUFFALO SAUCE & 50G CAESAR DRESSING

1236 cal per week

"I'VE BLOWN MY DIET"

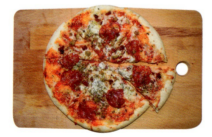

1X DOMINOS SMALL ITALIAN STYLE CRUST PEPPERONI PIZZA

1085 cal per week

Why You Shouldn't Log Exercise

Although we track and log our caloric intake, exercise is a different animal altogether. When exercise is logged in your app, the calories you theoretically burn will be added back into your daily budget. Add exercise manually, or your *Lose It!* premium membership enables the app to sync with activity trackers like Fitbit, Apple Watch, Misfit, Garmin, MapMyFitness, Runkeeper, and Strava, which do it for you.

We know calories in and out are most important for body composition goals, but we've also learned it will never be an exact science. When the correct activity factor is used to calculate your TDEE, your average daily calorie expenditure is accounted for. If you are considering connecting your wearable to *Lose It!*, please take the following into consideration:

Inaccuracy of Activity Trackers and Wearables

Activity trackers can be beneficial for goal setting, monitoring heart rate, and boosting daily NEAT levels; however, they have a large margin of error – especially when calculating burned calories. Stanford Medicine researchers who tested seven commercial fitness tracking devices under various conditions found that NONE had an accurate measure of calories burned.

The most accurate device was off by around 27%, and the least accurate was off by 93% [105,106]. Besides the lack of precision, using these tools can increase the risk of developing obsessive tracking of "calorie burn" and activity levels.

Inaccuracy of Self-Reporting

Studies have also shown pretty significant discrepancies between self-reported and actual calorie intake and exercise output. We tend to underreport food intake and over report exercise. Subjects in one study under-reported food intake by an average of 47%, and they over-reported physical activity by an average of 51% [105]. Food items with an adverse health image (cakes, sweets, and "junk food") are more likely to be under-reported, while those with a positive health image are more likely to be over-reported (fruits and vegetables) [107]. Women, overweight and obese individuals are more likely to under-report food than men [107].

Remember: Perfection Rarely Exists

Some days you might be 15g over on carbs and a bit short on protein. It's nearly impossible to weigh everything perfectly, or know *exactly* how many calories or grams of protein, carbs, and fats are in your food. If you finish the day with your macronutrients perfect, but calories are way over or under, it's important to note that the FDA has rounding rules for calories, proteins, carbs, and fats that can offset calculations by 10-15 calories.

The FDA also permits the total calories listed on food labels to equal the sum of carbohydrates, proteins, and fats, minus the calories from dietary fiber and sugar alcohols. Although, both still contain calories. This is essentially an incentive for food manufacturers to add more dietary fiber to their products. You'll often see the term "net carbohydrates" listed on labels. Net carbohydrates is a reflection of the total carbohydrate minus the dietary fiber. This is another arbitrary definition, which isn't all that useful for most of us, except for those who actually need to monitor their blood sugar levels more acutely.

Between user error in tracking, errors in measuring food, and FDA laws, this isn't an exact science. But, even in its flaws, macro-tracking is still one of the most efficient and effective ways to change your body composition and feel your best.

Instead of worrying about being absolutely "perfect" day in and out, look at weekly averages and trends with your nutrition in relation to your progress.

How to Use a Food Scale

If you don't want to doubt every single thing you eat down to the last tablespoon of peanut butter- weigh it! Weighing your food gives you a very accurate picture of how much you're eating and what portion sizes should look like, and it's relatively easy in the grand scheme of food prep and eating healthy. It also saves a lot of time and water not having to wash all those measuring utensils, always a huge plus! I know there are many food scales with different materials, pricing, and features to match. Fancy isn't necessary, but feel free to do your research and find a scale that works for your needs and budget.

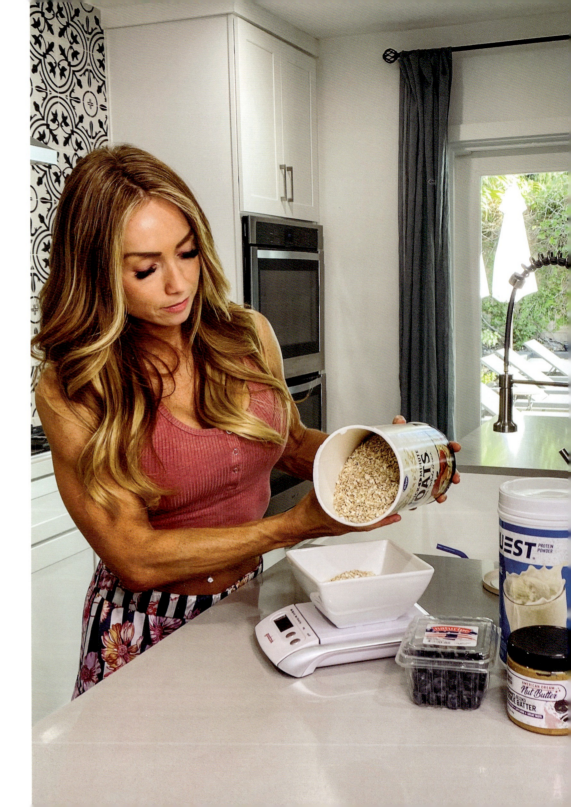

Download *Lose It!* http://fbuy.me/v/breannefreeman

Weigh Any Food

Due to fluctuations in water content after cooking, it's best to weigh your food raw, before cooking:

- Place your mixing bowl on the food scale.
- First, zero out the scale by using the "tare" button or the corresponding key. If the recipe you're using calls for measurement in g, mL, oz., or fl. oz., be sure the scale value matches.
- Add the first ingredient to your bowl.
- Zero out the food scale again.
- Add the second ingredient and repeat this process until you've added every ingredient.

Reverse Weigh Oils, Condiments, and Sauces

You might have a hot skillet that needs a bit of oil or a giant bowl of salad with no dressing that won't fit on your scale. Instead of dirtying another dish weighing your oils, condiments, or other toppings, weigh it in reverse. This method works best when you don't need as much precision. If you need a tiny serving, like one teaspoon of oil, I wouldn't recommend this method:

- Place the entire bottle of oil on the food scale.
- Zero-out the scale.
- Remove the bottle and add the oil to the pan, slowly.
- Place the bottle back on the scale. The number on the scale will be negative and tell you how much oil is "missing" from the bottle. That's how much you used.

Calculate Macronutrients Per Serving

Say you made a giant pot of Spicy Beef Mac and Cheese as part of your meal prep this week. It can be challenging to eyeball even servings. So here's how it's done:

- Place a large container on the food scale and zero out the scale.
- Transfer the recipe in its entirety to the large container. Note the recipe's total weight. For example, let's say the recipe weighs 2,000g.
- Add all the ingredients as a recipe in your *Lose It!* app and set the number of servings you want to dish out. If the entire recipe has 3,000 total calories, you could have six 500-calorie servings, ten 300-calorie servings, etc.
- The weight of your servings will depend on how many servings you want in step 3. If you go with the six 500-calorie servings, you would simply divide the 2,000g by six, and there you have it—each serving is 333g.
- You can divide the recipe into portions right away by transferring 333g into six containers or write a note on the large container and weigh each portion before reheating.

Pro Tip: If you weigh the pot or dish you're cooking with beforehand, you can weigh the entire pot without transferring the food to a large container. It might help to place a potholder or cloth on top of the food scale, so you don't have to wait for the pot to completely cool.

Success Story

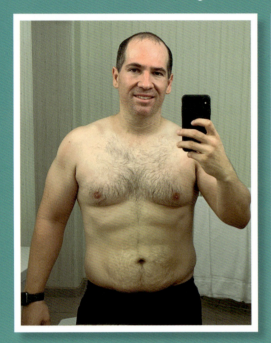
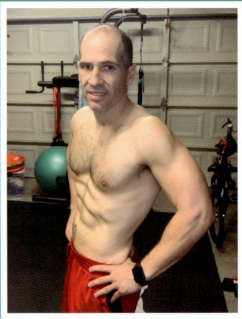

"I dropped 50 pounds in the first four months"

Ten years ago, I lost 125 pounds. That was a crazy eight months of my life. Like many, I enjoy exercising regularly, but the extreme diet regimen I followed was a struggle to maintain. I became diet-fatigued and just tried to eat "healthy" without a goal or plan. Eventually, half of the weight I lost crept back on, I was unhappy, and in the worst shape I had been in over a decade. This isn't the reality you want to face with five little ones running circles around you, plus one on the way.

I wanted change, but the thought of jumping back into my old diet kept me from moving forward. I was looking for a healthy lifestyle I could maintain, not a "quick fix," and Breanne's online fat loss challenge couldn't have come at a better time. I wanted to learn her macros-based nutrition plan, so I jumped on the opportunity. The moment I finished reading through the nutrition and workout materials is when everything changed. I knew exactly what and how much to eat to reach my goal using the calorie and macro formulas provided. This simple approach to nutrition provided the freedom I needed to get creative in the kitchen, cook meals my whole family loves, and even enjoy a glass of wine without guilt or blowing my goals.

I dropped 50 pounds in the first four months following this flexible nutrition plan coupled with four days of weight training every week. What's even better is I added strength and muscle in the process!

It's been over a year since that challenge and I can confidently say I'm in the best shape of my life. An unexpected by-product of this journey is learning the impact my transformation has made on others. Three close friends who have also struggled with their weight recently got in better shape and improved their health. I didn't know it, but they told me I was their inspiration. Knowing I've inspired others makes me happy, proud, and inspired to keep going.

- Lawrence Cortez

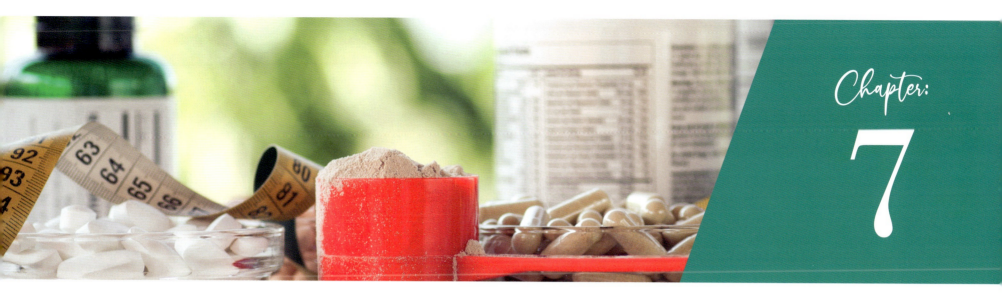

Supplements Worth Taking

The supplement business has become convoluted these days, with magic pills claiming to fix your weight problems, balance your hormones, boost your mood, improve your joints, and even satiate your hunger. These miracle supplements usually have a hefty price tag to match their hefty promises, and navigating fact from fiction can be an expensive headache. Only a few of these supplements have sufficient research to back up their claims, and I'm sure you want to save your hard-earned cash for the tried and true options. The following provides supplementation suggestions to improve health, boost fat loss, and increase muscle gain rates. The key is to remember that healthy habits are most important for meeting your weight-loss and muscle goals. Supplements can help you fill in some gaps, but they cannot replace a solid diet and exercise routine. It's also important to note that if you take any medications, always consult your healthcare professional before adding any supplement, as there may be unwanted interactions.

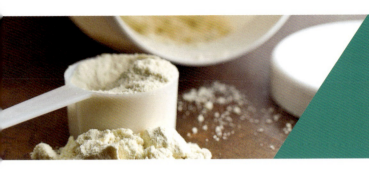

Protein Powder

I have placed a large emphasis in this guide on the importance of sufficient protein to reach your body composition goals, so it should come as no surprise that a protein supplement tops the tried and true supplement list. As you may recall from Chapter 2, whey is an ideal protein when it comes to quality and leucine content. **Getting enough daily protein can be a challenge when eating only whole foods, so adding a high-quality protein powder, like whey, is a convenient, effective way to reach daily protein targets. Whey protein (great any time of day), casein protein (best before bed), and vegan protein powders including soy, pea, and brown rice protein are all great options.**

A typical scoop of protein powder contains 25-30g of protein. Different brands and protein sources contain variable amounts of carbohydrates and fats as well. For a quick and easy protein dose, mix the powder with water or blend it into smoothies and drinks. For a more satisfying meal, mix protein powder into yogurt or milk, and add some fat – peanut butter is a personal favorite. A small piece of fruit and a fiber powder can make for a thick smoothie with a lot of nutrition. I've included a variety of tasty recipes in Chapter 12 using protein powders I know you'll enjoy.

While no supplements can replace a good, hearty meal, sometimes life can leave us in a pinch. Meal Replacement Powders, related to protein powders, are useful to hold you over until your next whole food meal. They typically contain a mixture of protein, carbohydrates, fat, fiber, and micronutrients. While these products should never make up a majority of your diet, they can provide convenience and a quick meal for busy individuals. Likewise, protein bars are a convenient option for those struggling to meet their daily protein needs. The best options will have a minimum of 40% calories from protein and provide at least 5g of fiber. Many bars today are a great "safe food" for those with a nagging sweet tooth, see Chapter 4 for a refresher on safe foods. Busy athletes often have trouble meeting their calorie and nutrient requirements and protein bars provide a quick, convenient source of calories and nutrients.

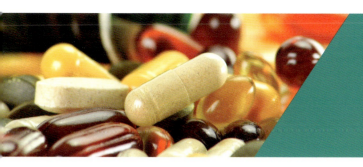

Multivitamin & Mineral

If you follow the *6 Rules for Complete Micronutrition* in Chapter 2, multivitamin and mineral supplementation may not be necessary. **Since eating a nutritionally optimal diet can be challenging, especially when following a calorie deficit diet for fat loss, a daily multivitamin and mineral can fill important nutrient gaps** [108]. For example, a zinc deficiency may reduce testosterone levels, and several other vitamins are important in regulating metabolic pathways [109,110]. It has been shown that multivitamin and mineral supplementation may help decrease hunger levels when trying to reduce calories [111]. Filling any potential nutrient gap is a simple great strategy to optimize health and fat loss goals.

Since they can only cram so much into tiny multivitamin and mineral pills, some individuals might need additional nutrients beyond what they provide. This varies by person and typically includes calcium, magnesium, iron, vitamin D, and zinc [108,112].

>> Women and aging populations can usually benefit from additional vitamin D and and/or calcium supplementation [113, 114].
>> Individuals with celiac disease can usually benefit from additional folate, vitamin B12, vitamin D, and calcium supplementation [109].
>> Those following a vegan diet might benefit from vitamin B12, vitamin D, omega fatty acids, and zinc.

It's also just as important to note that in certain people, vitamin supplementation can do more harm than good. For example, those with a history of kidney stones may have a higher risk of recurrence if they use calcium supplements [115]. A multivitamin and mineral supplement is best taken with a meal as there are likely to be nutrients or other factors found in the food being eaten that will improve absorption. Vitamins A, D and K are fat-soluble and are best absorbed with a fat containing meal. As always, talk to your doctor before adding any supplement to your daily routine.

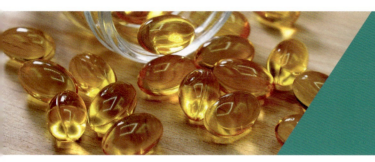

Omega-3 Fish Oil

If you recall from Chapter 2, Essential Fatty Acids (EFA) must be consumed through diet and provide many health benefits. Except for those cultures that eat fatty fish regularly, the intake of EFA's, particularly Omega-3 fatty acids, is generally low in the North American diet [116]. **Being deficient in omega-3 can lead to fatigue, poor cognition and memory, depression, and an increased risk of cardiovascular disease [116,117]. Collectively, these negative effects may impact your muscle building and fat loss goals.** While fish oils are absorbed more effectively from fatty fish, you can boost omega-3 intake by consuming more grass-fed meats, free-range egg yolk, flaxseed, walnuts, chia seeds, and spinach. Supplementation with 2-6g of omega-3 per day ensures minimum daily requirements are met [118]. Individuals under 160 pounds should be ok with the lower dose and those heavier should shoot for more.

Note: Controversy over omega-3 supplementation surfaced after a study suspected an increased risk for prostate cancer. Dietary consumption of fish or fish oil was not actually assessed in this study, and if this were true, populations with high omega-3 fatty acid intake should also have a relatively high risk for prostate cancer; this does not seem to be the case [115,119,120]. Recent research has confirmed omega-3 fatty acids have no effect on prostate cancer. In fact, higher levels of omega-3 have protective and prostate cancer lowering effects in men [121].

Sleep Aids

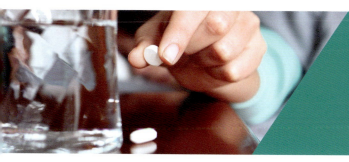

Sleep is an extremely underrated weight management tool and general health promoter. Sleep is the time our body heals from the day's stress, including our exercise regimen. Without enough sleep, both muscle building and fat loss can be hard. The effects of sleep deprivation are not completely understood, but sleeping five hours or less is associated with an increase in obesity among men by 3.7 times, and a 2.3-fold increase in obesity among women, compared to those who sleep seven to eight hours per night [145]. Essentially, when we don't get enough sleep, our bodies want/need more energy. As a result, it produces more ghrelin (the hormone that makes us hungry) and decreases leptin (the hormone that helps us feel full). A systematic review of eleven studies concluded poor sleep patterns resulted in an average of 385 extra calories consumed per day [122]! So, don't just aim for six to eight hours, aim for six to eight *quality* hours. There are many ways to improve sleep without supplementation.

>> Consume carbohydrates before bedtime. This raises serotonin levels which promotes sleep.

>> Set a sleep schedule to go to bed and wake up the same time each day.

>> Eliminate alcohol and stimulants, like caffeine, that may interfere with sleep. If you are on medications that act as stimulants, such as decongestants or asthma inhalers, ask your doctor when they should best be taken to help minimize any effect on sleep.

>> Make your sleeping environment comfortable. Things like temperature, lighting, and noise should be controlled to make the bedroom conducive to falling and staying asleep.

>> Shut electronic devices off one to two hours before sleep.

While the above scenarios are ideal, they're not always possible. Therefore, melatonin supplementation is worth considering. A standard dose ranges from 1-10mg per day, and the optimal dose has not been formally established [123]. Many find small doses are sufficient. Other sleep supplements like Theanine (found in tea), dosed at 100-200mg before sleep, can quiet the mind and soothe anxiety. Gaba Amino Butyric Acid (GABA), dosed at 500mg an hour before sleep, is a relaxation and anti-anxiety supplement that helps some sleep. Lastly, 5-HTP, dosed at 50-100mg up to three times per day, including one hour before sleep, can improve sleep, mood, and carbohydrate cravings.

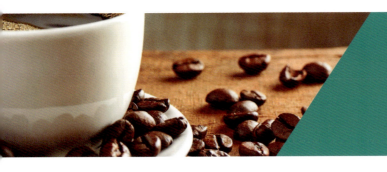

Caffeine

Caffeine, a natural alkaloid, is arguably the supplement used most around the world. Common caffeine sources include the kola nut, cacao bean, yerba mate, guarana berry, roasted coffee beans, and tea leaves. **Evidence shows it boosts cognitive function, increases energy expenditure and strength, prolongs fatigue, and boosts acute fat oxidation during and after exercise** [124, 125].

For those with fat loss goals, caffeine has a beneficial effect on energy balance [126–128]. Supplementing with 600mg per day can boost calorie burn by an extra 100 calories per day. As long as calories are controlled, this could result in one pound of fat loss per month. Research has also shown caffeine has an appetite reducing effect, and therefore, can reduce calorie intake [128]. Daily caffeine intake at 5mg per kg of body weight per day (300mg for a 132 pound/60 kg woman) can prevent weight regain following a fat loss diet [128,129].

The effect caffeine has on exercise performance makes it a beneficial supplement for muscle gain goals as well. Most experience increased muscular endurance and can perform more reps with a given weight [130]. One study did find a small increase in the maximum amount a woman could bench press with caffeine [131]. A healthy daily caffeine intake varies per person. For those with the primary goal of fat loss or alertness, supplement with a low dose of 1-2mg per kg of body weight before doing cardio. To maximize strength performance, a much higher dose of 3-6mg per kg of body weight can be utilized up to two times per week. It's not advised to exceed 400-600mg a day. To put this into perspective, a cup of coffee is about 60mg, 12oz of diet soda is about 30mg, a standard caffeine pill contains 200mg, and some energy drinks can contain up to 400mg. The more frequently high doses of caffeine are consumed, the less effective it becomes, since the body develops a tolerance. Always use caffeine responsibly to avoid unwanted side effects like elevated blood pressure, feeling nervous, jittery, anxious, gastrointestinal distress, and insomnia.

Green Tea (ECGC) with Caffeine

Green Tea's active ingredient epigallocatechin-3-gallate, or ECGC, is another thermogenic compound you can add to your supplement arsenal. **When combined with caffeine, ECGC can increase calorie burn by four percent when compared to caffeine intake alone** [132]. Therefore, taken prior to exercise, EGCG with caffeine can be an effective tool to enhance fat-loss. The recommended dose is 125-250mg of EGCG with around 100mg of caffeine taken up to three times per day. Herbal supplements all tend to be dosed differently, but each should indicate how much EGCG is present.

Yohimbine HCL with Caffeine

Yohimbine is a supplement derived from Yohimbe Tree Bark. It is not a thermogenic that boosts calorie burn like caffeine or ECGC. Instead, it has been shown to enhance fat loss [132,133] and decrease appetite by increasing adrenaline (also known as epinephrine). It can also inhibit the processes that suppress fat loss.

In an ideal fat loss scenario, epinephrine binds to beta receptors instead of alpha receptors on fat cells. From a fat loss perspective, alpha receptors are "bad" and beta receptors are "good." Yohimbine inhibits the alpha-2 receptors, leaving more beta receptors available for epinephrine to bind to [134]. Essentially, it is disabling the fat loss inhibitor. A secondary effect of yohimbine is an increase of blood flow into these fat cells, which assists fat loss. Combining yohimbine with caffeine enhances these effects. "Bad" alpha receptors are typically found within stubborn fat, such as the hip areas of women and abdominal areas of men. This is why it is suggested to wait until body fat levels are lower (women under 20% and men under 15%) before adding yohimbine supplementation.

Yohimbine can be found as Yohimbine HCL, a synthetic form, and Yohimbe Bark, an herbal form. The herbal form tends to be dosed poorly and causes negative side-effects like increased heart rate, anxiety, and blood pressure. Therefore, yohimbine HCL is the preferred use to minimize these effects. It's important to note that insulin can disrupt Yohimbine HCL's effects, so it's ideally taken either after an overnight fast, three to four hours after a meal when insulin levels have decreased, or one hour before low or moderate-intensity cardio. If lifting weights first, work backwards based on the length of your session. For example, take yohimbine HCL immediately before a one-hour weighted workout.

The recommended dose is 0.2mg per kg of body weight. This means a 150 pound individual would take 13.5mg. Since yohimbine HCL is usually dosed 2.5mg per pill, 5-6 pills of 12.5-15mg is needed. *Begin with a half dose to assess tolerance before increasing.*

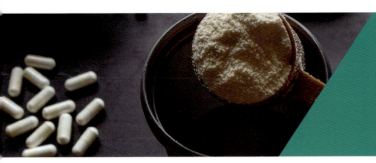

Creatine Monohydrate

Creatine is the most researched supplement in the world, with more than 700 human studies. The International Society of Sports Nutrition has deemed creatine to be the safest and most effective ergogenic aid, yet confusion among the general population still lingers around its use, results, and safety.

Creatine is produced in the liver, kidneys, and pancreas and stored in the skeletal muscle of the body as phosphocreatine. People also consume creatine through red meat and seafood, which is why vegetarians may have lower amounts of creatine in their bodies [123, 135]. Phosphocreatine is the fuel source primarily utilized for short duration, high-intensity work such such as heavy weight training and sprinting. Supplementing with creatine simply increases phosphocreatine stores to provide more available energy for high-intensity work.

Across all ages and genders, creatine supplementation has demonstrated increased strength, power, muscular endurance, high-intensity exercise performance, muscle, and strength [136, 137]. Benefits of supplementing with creatine go beyond exercise performance. Creatine also helps offset the loss of bone density and muscle mass in older women [138], has shown to help with some types of depression [139], provides neuroprotective properties [140], and produces several potential benefits for pregnancy.

Many women steer clear of creatine for fear of unwanted weight gain. While it does cause some water retention, water is drawn into the muscle where you want it, not under the skin [141]. Due to differences in total body muscle mass, this averages around one pound for women and two pounds or more for men [136], which is lost with discontinued use.

There are two creatine dosing methods that can increase muscular creatine stores by 20-40% [140, 142]. The first is a loading phase, a larger dose of 20-25g throughout the day for five to seven days, followed with a maintenance intake of 3-10g per day. The second method is a simple daily dose of 3-5g. Individuals with greater muscle mass are likely to benefit from the higher dose of either method [143]. Creatine in tandem with a carbohydrate increases uptake and muscular retention [138]. The time of day you supplement with creatine is much less important than consistency in every-day use [141].

Beta-alanine with Creatine

Beta-alanine is a relatively newer supplement, but solid research backs its ability to boost exercise duration, and performance in maximal-intensity activities lasting up to 10 minutes [144]. This includes weight training, most forms of HIIT, and 400m to the 1600m running. Beta-alanine works by elevating carnosine levels in the muscle. Carnosine buffers the acid-induced burning sensation within the muscles during these types of training activities.

Beta-alanine is dosed at 3.2-4.6g per day, divided into doses of 2g or less for at least two weeks, with greater benefits seen after 4 weeks. Beta-alanine may be even more effective at increasing strength, power, and muscle mass when used with creatine. In one study, the combination of 10g of creatine and 3.2g of beta-alanine per day enabled more training output to be performed.

Additional training volume in the long-term leads to greater gains in strength and muscle hypertrophy. Since women and vegetarians tend to have lower levels of muscle carnosine and creatine, they might find a greater benefit when supplementing with both.

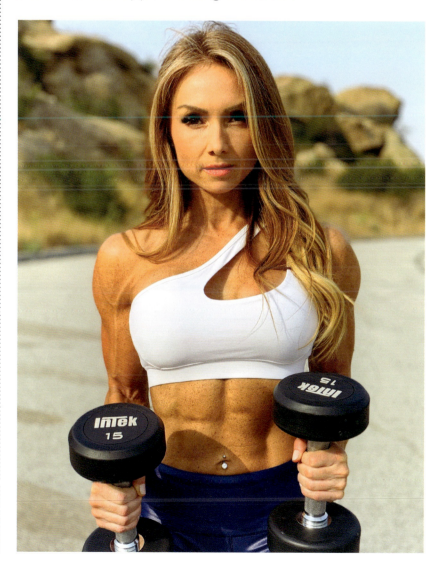

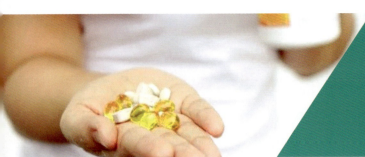

L-Citrulline

Of the many supplements claiming to improve performance and gains over time, l-citrulline is one of few that has plenty of scientific support in its favor [145-148]. When exercising, your muscles need oxygen for performance. Oxygen delivery can be optimized by increasing blood arginine levels which boost nitric oxide (NO), and therefore, increase blood vessel diameter (also known as vasodilation). More blood flow leads to more efficient oxygen delivery, as well as better uptake of glucose and amino acids into the muscle.

While l-arginine is the precursor for the synthesis of NO, l-citrulline is actually more efficient at increasing blood arginine levels than supplementing with l-arginine directly. This is because it metabolizes differently and enters the bloodstream faster, which gives a more efficient increase of blood flow and oxygen to the muscles. Supplementation with l-citrulline can also reduce blood pressure in adults with pre-/hypertension, improve muscle and metabolic health in older populations, and boost immunity. Another added bonus is its antioxidant and anti-inflammatory effects [148, 149]. L-citrulline is dosed 4-10g before workout. Unfortunately, many companies either underdose in their pre workout formulas, or hide the true amount within a "proprietary blend." Similar to caffeine, our bodies can build a tolerance to l-citrulline, therefore, cycle on and off periodically as you notice its effects diminishing.

Putting Your Supplementation Plan Together

General Health Supplements
- **Protein Powder:** high quality whey or a vegan blend as needed for daily protein goals.
- **Multivitamin & Mineral:** as needed to fill nutrient gaps in diet.
- **Omega-3 Fish Oil:** 2g per day if fatty fish is not consumed regularly.
- **Sleep Aids:** As needed.

Muscle Gain Supplements
- **Caffeine:** 3-6mg per kg body weight pre workout, 1-2x per week for strength and performance.
- **Creatine:** 5g per day.
- **Beta-alanine:** 3.2- 4.6g per day, divided into two doses and paired with creatine pre workout.
- **L-Citrulline:** 4-10g taken pre workout.

For a 150 lb person: 200mg Caffeine, 5g Creatine, 2g (x 2) Beta-alanine, up to 10g L-Citrulline.

Fat Loss Supplements
- **Caffeine:** 1-2mg per kg body weight pre workout for general alertness, cardio, and fat loss.
- **Green Tea (EGCG):** 125-250mg paired with caffeine pre workout.
- **Yohimbine HCL:** 0.2mg per kg of body weight one hour before cardio, on an empty stomach. Only to be used as an advanced stubborn fat loss strategy. Begin with a half dose to assess tolerance before increasing.

For a 150 lb person: 70mg Caffeine, 250mg EGCG, up to 15mg Yohimbine HCL.

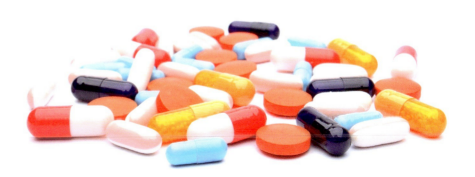

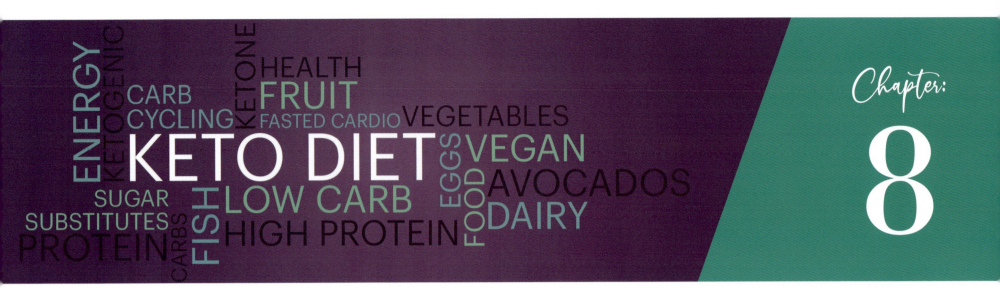

Chapter: 8

Other Nutrition Hot Topics

The ever-changing nutrition landscape has made it difficult to understand today's trending hot topics. From fasted cardio to Keto, sugar substitutes, dairy, and gluten; without a doubt, you have questions! This chapter will help clear the path through today's maze of misinformation with the research to back it up.

ARE SUGAR SUBSTITUTES HEALTH HAZARDS?

With concerns about obesity on the rise, sugar substitutes, also known as non-nutritive sweeteners (NNS), offer the satisfaction of satiating a sweet tooth without the calories or metabolic effects of pure sugar. Many are made naturally, usually extracted from plants, while some are made synthetically. As the name indicates, non-nutritive sweeteners have zero calories while sugar has four calories per gram. A 12-ounce can of soda that contains 40g of sugar provides 160 unsatiating calories- so eliminating these foods should make weight loss an easier endeavor, right?

Today, NNS remains a point of controversy. Some believe that they actually cause weight gain and metabolic diseases. Let's take a look at the research, starting with obesity and weight loss:

> A meta-analysis of 15 randomized trials showed that substituting sugar with NNS modestly reduced body weight, fat mass, and waist circumference among people who are overweight or obese [150].

> Subsequent studies found that drinking 24 ounces of diet soda per day leads to significantly greater weight loss and less hunger over a 12-week period than drinking 24 ounces of water. This resulted in maintaining greater weight loss over a year-long follow-up [151, 152].

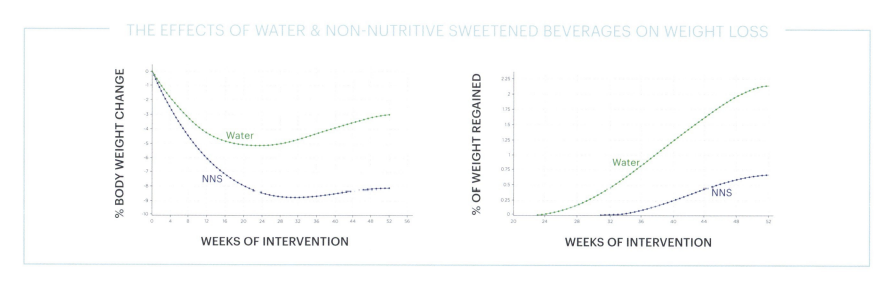

THE EFFECTS OF WATER & NON-NUTRITIVE SWEETENED BEVERAGES ON WEIGHT LOSS

Master Your Macros

So, should we recommend diet soda over water? Certainly not, but these studies show it is definitely an improvement over sugar-sweetened beverages and that it does not hinder weight loss.

So, if NNS help with weight loss efforts, how do we explain the link to obesity? Researchers have concluded that obese people simply tend to consume more diet beverages and foods in attempt to lose weight [153]. This doesn't mean the sweeteners caused the weight gain. Additionally, it has been found that people who consume more NNS also tend to live unhealthier lifestyles; like eating more calories overall and exercising less [154].

Other NNS findings worth pointing out:
>> Some studies have shown that replacing regular soda with diet soda can reduce fat around the liver [155, 156].
>> Current data shows that carbonated drinks have not been found to make acid reflux or heartburn worse. However, the research is mixed, and more experimental studies are needed [157, 158].
>> Most of the research on NNS and diet soda has found no evidence it causes cancer [159].
>> 50 of 60 studies reported either no effects or reductions in appetite and food intake with consumption of NNS [160].
>> The effects on the glycemic control are thought to be tied to an individual's gut microbiome. Consuming NSS on an empty stomach could have a more pronounced effect [161, 162]. To what extent this effect outweighs the potential benefit of losing weight remains unclear.

We do know that studies are consistently showing that non-nutritive sweeteners help with weight loss when they replace sugar, because they help dieters reduce caloric intake without depriving themselves of sweets. And losing weight is an established method of reducing the risk of Type 2 diabetes and improving insulin sensitivity [163]. I wouldn't suggest replacing water with diet soda, but the choice is yours to enjoy diet drinks and NNS without worrying about unintentionally hindering weight loss, at least as long as you do not compensate for it by eating more calories from other food.

Safe NNS intake guidelines offered by the FDA:

		FDA safe intake levels (mg/kg body weight)	Safe # of packets for a 132-pound adult
Artificial NNS	Acesulfame & Potassium (Ace-K)	15	23
	Advantame	32.8	4,920
	Aspartame	50	75
	Neotame	0.3	23
	Saccharin	15	45
	Sucralose	5	23
Natural NNS	Stevia extract	4*	9*
	Monk Fruit extract	Unknown	Unknown

*Stevia is a newer sweetener, so more research is needed to determine safe intake levels. Source: [164]

IS DAIRY UNHEALTHY?

There are various reasons people make the decision to cut dairy from their diet. Some are lactose intolerant and lack the enzymes to digest the sugars specific to dairy. Others believe it causes acne, inflammation and weight gain. The reality is, consuming dairy can be beneficial on many levels. With critical micronutrients, like zinc and B12, calcium and vitamin D, sufficient dairy intake helps the development of bone density in childhood, and it prevents bone density loss later in life. Also, a review of 52 clinical trials found significantly positive data indicating dairy as an *anti-inflammatory* in humans. Fermented products were shown to be particularly anti-inflammatory, and those with metabolic disorders seemed to benefit more. However, those with dairy allergies had a pro-inflammatory effect, which shouldn't seem surprising [165].

Weight loss from dairy elimination is often due to how it was consumed before, how much, and in what form. So, if pizza, mac and cheese, and grilled cheese sandwiches were your go-to meals, you should now understand the reason for said weight loss. The evidence shows that regular consumption of dairy, like milk, yogurt, Greek yogurt, kefir, and cheese are associated with a reduced risk of childhood obesity and greater fat loss rates [166,167]. Since dairy proteins are a high-quality source of Branched Chain Amino Acids (BCAA), they're excellent for muscle growth and preservation while dieting. The presence of active cultures in yogurt also acts as a probiotic to improve gut health [168]. The good news is for some lactose intolerant individuals, cutting back on your overall intake, or consuming dairy products along with other foods (such as cereal with milk instead of ice cream by itself) may be enough to ease symptoms.

IS CARB-CYCLING IDEAL FOR FAT LOSS?

"Carb cycling" has gotten more public attention than it deserves. The idea that you can somehow "trick your body" or "keep your metabolism guessing" by cycling through high carb, moderate carb, and low carb days has no basis in the scientific literature. Ultimately, fat loss will be determined by energy balance throughout the week, so arbitrarily increasing and decreasing carb intake throughout the week will not provide any extra metabolic benefits. For example, setting Monday as your high carb day, Tuesday as your moderate carb day, and Wednesday as your low carb day, has no metabolic advantage from a fat loss perspective. It certainly is just as effective as having an equal, moderate carb intake on all three days.

IS FRUIT FATTENING?

When was the last time you heard anyone say, "You know... all those blueberries are what packed on those last 10 pounds!" Sounds silly, right? Know when you eat a piece of fruit, like a banana, your body is getting other things out of it besides sugar, like potassium, magnesium, vitamin C, vitamin B6, and fiber that your body needs to stay healthy. The sugar in fruit is called fructose, a slow releasing sugar that the body converts into glucose before it can effectively use it. Breaking down vitamins, minerals, fiber, and fructose all slows down the digestion process, making fruit very different than consuming a piece of candy or a can of soda that has very few nutrients. As long as your overall calories are aligned with your goals, enjoying an apple a day will not result in weight gain.

ARE GLUTEN-FREE DIETS HEALTHIER?

The term "gluten" refers to a collection of proteins found in grains. Gluten-free diets are essential for patients with celiac disease, wheat allergies, or a non-celiac gluten sensitivity (NCGS). Gluten related disorders, however, are uncommon and only impact around 5% of the global population. While those sensitive to gluten clearly benefit from following a gluten-free diet, there is currently little to no evidence that suggests eliminating gluten will help with weight-loss, cognitive function, health or performance in those who do not suffer with a gluten-related disorder when compared to gluten-containing whole-food-based diets [66]. On the contrary, there are actually significant drawbacks to following the gluten-free diet for those not afflicted with gluten allergies. Gluten-free products tend to be significantly more expensive, and gluten-free grain products like breads, cereals, and crackers are also often lower in fiber, iron, zinc, and potassium, while higher in fat and calories than their gluten-containing counterparts [169]. If you aren't sure whether gluten affects you in a negative way, please consult your doctor. But if you're not affected, some gluten in your diet can be advantageous.

IS KETO THE KEY TO FAT LOSS?

If you don't know someone who's on the ketogenic diet, you soon will. Keto is a diet strategy that calls for 55-60% calories from fat, 30-35% from protein and 5-10% from carbohydrates. When calories are matched, weight loss in pounds will be higher when following keto, but the difference is explained by water weight loss due to depleted glycogen stores [170]. As soon as carbs are consumed, glycogen is restored and lost water weight returns.

There are also some potential negative side effects to the Keto diet. They include reduced exercise performance, reduced libido, hepatic steatosis (fatty liver), hypoproteinemia (abnormally low level of protein in the blood), kidney stones, loss of muscle (reduced protein and carbs), constipation (lack of fiber), deficiency of many vitamins and minerals, and the latest discovery: "keto crotch" [171]. Keto crotch symptoms include strong smelling vaginal odor and white discharge- yikes! Significant increases in saturated fat intake have also linked keto to increases in LDL cholesterol and heart disease with increased all-cause mortality [172].

Unless under the recommendation and supervision of a doctor, extreme dietary measures, like Keto, can be unhealthy and unnecessary. Stick to a reasonable calorie deficit, include a variety of whole foods, and your desired fat loss can be achieved without the extremes.

DOES FASTED CARDIO BOOST FAT LOSS?

Fasted cardio is a fancy way to describe exercising on an empty stomach. The theory behind it is that when you haven't eaten for an extended period of time, especially carbohydrates, your glycogen levels are low so your body is more likely to turn to stored fat to supply the energy needed for fuel. When calories and macronutrients are controlled, several studies have shown no differences in fat loss between fasted and fed cardio groups [173–176].

Findings from a 2011 study provided some very interesting insights. When measuring respiratory exchange ratio (RER), an indicator of whether carbohydrate or fat is being metabolized for fuel, results found that the body's main fuel source during fasted cardio were fatty acids. However, fat oxidation shifted in favor of the fed cardio participants when measured

Master Your Macros

12 and 24 hours post exercise session [177]. The authors concluded that over long periods, exercising after breakfast could be more effective than fasted exercise for fat loss.

While the research will likely go back and forth on this subject, I believe the differences to be minimal in the grand scheme of energy balance and fat loss. When fat loss is the goal, focus first on creating a meaningful caloric deficit rather than worrying about exercising in fed or fasted states. If your performance suffers on an empty stomach, try a small carb and protein snack 30-45 minutes prior to a workout. Improved performance should lead to a better workout, and a better workout should lead to better results. If getting cardio done first thing in the morning before a meal is preferable, that is reasonable as well.

ARE HIGH PROTEIN DIETS BAD FOR KIDNEYS AND BONES?

Some people worry that too much protein might overtax their kidney, liver, or bones. The kidneys and liver produce and process a nitrogen-containing waste, urea, that is excreted in the urine. Now it's true that eating a lot of protein will increase urea. For most healthy individuals with regular kidney function, the research has consistently shown no negative side effects of high protein diets. In fact, in studies that compare low, moderate, and high protein diets, only the low protein diets showed a risk to bone health and decreased kidney function in healthy individuals [178, 179]. Considering high protein diets (1g per pound per day) have been associated with increased satiety, lower stress levels, less mood disturbance, and diet-related stress compared to moderate protein (0.7g per pound per day), consuming more protein in any diet is a highly recommended strategy [91].

DOES EATING MEAT REDUCE LIFESPAN?

Recent media headlines claim if you cut back on protein, you may live longer. It's hard to study longevity with accuracy. When just comparing vegetarians as a group to non-vegetarians in observational studies, vegetarians do indeed live longer, with a 12% lowered risk of dying from any cause compared to non-vegetarians. Vegetarians, however, also tend to have a higher education, exercise more, sleep more, smoke less, and drink less alcohol [180]. This means that when comparing vegetarians to non-vegetarians, we are also comparing highly educated, physically active, non-smokers to less educated, less active smokers. This makes it difficult for us to know if vegetarians live longer because of their diet or because of their lifestyle.

A 2017 meta-analysis took observational data from 130,000 vegetarians and 15,000 vegans, and compared them to a group of non-vegetarians. When lifestyle differences were adjusted, vegetarian diets did not result in an increased lifespan [173]. Another meta-analysis looking at cancer and heart disease among vegetarians came up with the same conclusion [173,174]. While the overall lifestyle adopted by vegetarians can help them live longer, the vegetarian diet itself does not get all the credit for those benefits. One thing is certain: maintaining a lower body mass index by slightly reducing total daily calories is a more likely life-extending practice [181].

Please note the topics of this chapter were provided to clarify some of today's nutrition hot topics based on current research. Ultimately, a nutrition plan that is healthy, enjoyable, and sustainable can look different for different people. Through your personal preferences and experiences, you can make the best decisions for yourself!

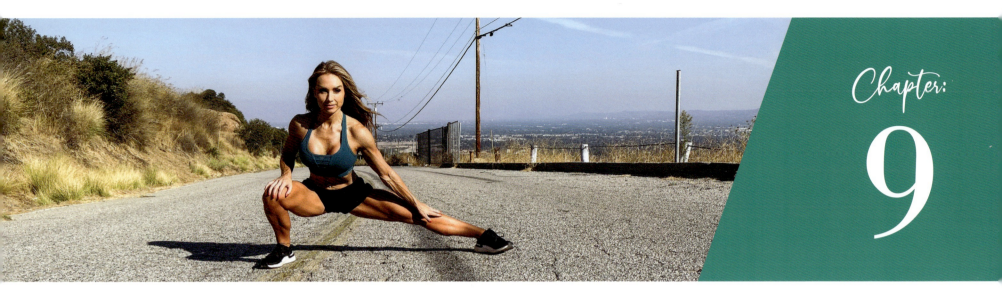

Navigating Your Journey: FAQ's

Changing your body composition can be a slow endeavor. Fat loss is slow and muscle gain is even slower. When you don't see immediate results, it can be tempting to second guess your method and make adjustments more frequently than you should. *Remember, calorie calculations are not an exact science. There are so many different variables that affect your energy balance,* so when self-coaching, it is extremely helpful to have basic guidelines. This Q&A will help you navigate the journey ahead.

Do You Have to Track Your Food Forever?

Losing fat and building muscle requires you to adopt and maintain a combination of new behaviors. This may turn into a constant nag repeating in your mind: Eat less. Eat better. Move more. Lift. You need to find ways to make unhealthy environments support your goals. Reframe how to react in a high-calorie environment. Re-prioritize time so weight loss and muscle building promoting behaviors fit in. Ugh!

I've spent a lot of time bouncing from diet to diet before discovering calorie and macro tracking and giving Flexible Dieting a go. We live in an environment where food is everywhere! Food is social, and it's too easy to overeat without realizing it. So, even after years of using *Lose It!*, I have found if I'm not tracking my calories I'm probably overdoing it. While calorie counting may be a tedious habit to start, it is worth it in the end! The length of time you track is up to you. Some can track for a year, build the knowledge about the foods they eat, and create the discipline it takes to maintain results. Others find food tracking a good and long-term accountability tool that keeps them, well, on track.

Are Your Calorie Calculations Too Low?

Did you calculate a daily calorie goal under 1,200? Calorie calculations under 1,200 probably aren't necessary for most people, but there are instances where it's perfectly fine. Petite women, around 5'2" and 110 pounds or lighter, who are fairly sedentary throughout the day, don't require as many calories as a larger, more active individual. Likewise, it shouldn't be necessary to drop below 22 calories per kg, or 10 calories per pound of current body weight per day. This equates to 1,200 calories for a 120 pound individual.

If you calculated a number you aren't comfortable with, make the adjustments necessary that work for you and your lifestyle. As long as you are eating fewer calories than your body requires daily, you will lose weight. Also know that the guidelines provided aren't hard targets. Individuals starting at a lower body fat percentage should diet slower to prevent muscle catabolism (see Chapter 3).

Do You Count All Carbs or "Net Carbs"?

The term 'net carbs' simply refers to carbs that are absorbed by the body. To calculate the net carbs in whole foods, subtract the fiber from the total number of carbs. To calculate the net carbs in processed foods, subtract the fiber and a portion of the sugar alcohols. This seems to be a fair representation of what is parroted around the internet fitness industry, but it also suggests fiber and sugar alcohols are calorie-free, which is incorrect.

Some fiber, while not digestible in the small intestine, is fermented in the colon, and that by-product provides energy. There are also many different types of sugar alcohols with calorie values ranging from 0.2-4 per gram. Determining which fibers and sugar alcohols provide calories and exactly how many is quite difficult. For simplicity, I recommend counting all carbs as four calories per gram. Ignore the net carb concept, otherwise you risk getting yourself in a pickle.

How Do You Measure Progress?

When dieting, there are many data points that help you measure progress. The scale, BMI, improved fitness levels, lower body fat percentage, better sleep, measurements, pictures, even compliments from others –so it's best not to rely on just one. When you've got multiple data points showing progress, know you are heading in the right direction.

Scale Weight & Body Mass Index (BMI)

Please remember the scale is just one data point among many ways to measure progress as you lose fat and build muscle. Similar to the BMI system, which estimates body fat based only on height and weight, most scales do not account for daily fluctuations in water weight and the possibility of building muscle while losing fat. Look at it this way: if you weigh an equal volume of fat and muscle, the muscle will outweigh fat by almost double. Therefore, if you gain five pounds of muscle and lose five pounds of fat you'll look much better, your clothes will fit better, you'll feel better, people will notice, but the scale might show "no progress" because your weight is the same. Therefore, if your goal is fat loss, an increase in weight due to an increase in muscle mass is a sign of progress, not a reason to lose motivation.

The scale can be a beneficial tool to shed light on what's happening long-term. If your goal is muscle gain and the scale is slowly going up without large increases in fat levels, you're on the right path. If your goal is fat loss, the scale should eventually reflect a decrease in weight even if muscle is being built simultaneously because fat loss happens much quicker than muscle gain. This is particularly true for advanced lifters whose rates of muscle gain are the slowest.

Since you will naturally fluctuate around five pounds over the course of a single day, remaining consistent when weighing yourself is important. The most accurate results would be first thing in the morning, before you eat or drink and after you go to the bathroom. Weigh yourself every day and calculate weekly averages for a more accurate depiction of progress. Here's an example of your morning weigh-ins:

> WK1 D1 – 155.4 pounds
> WK1 D2 - 154.2 pounds
> WK1 D3 – 155.8 pounds
> WK1 D4 – 155.2 pounds
> WK1 D5 - 153.6 pounds

From this set of five weigh-ins across the week, you would calculate the first weekly average to be 154.8 pounds. The next week, you would collect more weigh-ins:

> WK2 D1 – 154.0 pounds
> WK2 D2– 154.5 pounds
> WK2 D3 – 153.8 pounds
> WK2 D4 – 154.1 pounds
> WK2 D5 – 153.5 pounds
> WK2 D6 – 154.0 pounds

For this set of six weigh-ins, you would calculate the second weekly weight average to be 153.9 pounds. You've lost one pound, great work!

Over time, average weekly weigh-ins can help assess whether your bodyweight is trending up or down, which will help determine what is in line with your goal. Note that you do not need to weigh in every single day to get an average measurement, unless you find that convenient. Also, keep in mind that weigh-in fluctuations are completely normal. Variables like stress levels, water intake, sodium intake, carbohydrate intake, food volume, the menstrual cycle, and bowel movements can impact your body weight on a daily basis.

Measurements

Since scale weight really doesn't tell us that much about actual body composition, measurements are extremely helpful. Using a fabric tape measure, obtain these key bits of information: waist circumference, shoulders, glutes, chest, hips, thigh, biceps, and calves. Measure at the belly button / smallest site on your waist. For all other body parts, measure at the largest muscle site. Record both left and right measurements to track any asymmetries and correct for imbalances. As you lose fat, many of these measurements might decrease, even if muscle gain has occurred. To avoid fluctuations due to water retention, take waist measurements one to two times per month, on the same days each month and be consistent with the locations over time.

Body Fat Testing

While there are a variety of body fat testing methods, some are more accurate than others, but none are 100% accurate. Popular methods used today include skinfold calipers, bioelectrical impedance scales, hydrostatic weighing, air displacement plethysmography (Bod Pod), and dual-energy x-ray absorptiometry (DXA)- which is considered the gold standard. The more accurate the method, the more expensive and harder it is to come by. The important thing is to pick one method and stick with it to assess progress over time. Measurements, body weight, and body fat percentages can be tracked in your *Lose It!* app premium membership.
Get a free week of Lose It premium features at
http://fbuy.me/v/breannefreeman

Progress Pictures

Can be the most valuable tool of all! Because we are usually more concerned with achieving a certain look, scale or tape measurements can be less important. Since body composition changes can be harder to visually detect from week to week, take progress photos every one to two months wearing the same outfit, in the same room, with the same lighting. Standing normally, take three photos of yourself: one from the side, one from the front, and one from the back. No flexing, no sucking in. Another tip: look at your face. Fat loss often occurs there first, or at least it's noticed in the face, chin and neck area first. You won't notice this yourself from day to day, but other people will, and regular progress photos will make it apparent to you too. As a great bonus, visual evidence can be very motivating and validating.

Strength Changes

You're more likely to feel changes before you see them, so don't get discouraged in the short term. Ask yourself these questions: Can you train longer, lift heavier, or complete your exercises with more ease? Are you finding it easier to carry heavy groceries? Are your kids or pets getting lighter? These are good indicators you're building muscle! If your leggings, sports bras, jeans and t-shirts fit looser, you're making progress; keep it up!

Did You Set Up Your Calories & Macros Correctly?

After a full month of tracking your food on your plan, do a self-assessment to determine if progress is in line with your goal. How is your physique looking? Are body fat levels improving? Are strength levels improving? How is the number on the scale changing in response to your caloric intake?

SIGNS YOU'RE ON THE RIGHT PATH:

>> Your primary goal is fat loss
After one month you find that your waist circumference is down, your progress photos are looking leaner and tighter and your weekly bodyweight average is lower, the same, or similar (you could be adding a bit of muscle!), then you are on the right path. When we begin to diet and see results, it can be tempting to reduce calories even more to see even bigger results. The best-case scenario for our metabolism and mental sanity is to lose as much weight as possible while eating as much food as possible. Only when your progress begins to slow down or stall is the only time to adjust your intake - a little bit at a time. Make sure you give yourself enough time to see progress.

>> Your primary goal is muscle gain
If after one month the number on the scale is up, your waist circumference is lower or the same and you are getting stronger and noticing muscle definition in your progress photos, this is a good indicator you are on the right path.

>> Your primary goal is fat loss OR muscle gain
If after one month the number on the scale is the same or slightly up, but your waist circumference is down and your progress photos are looking leaner and more muscular, this is a good indicator you have built muscle while losing body fat.

SIGNS IT'S TIME TO ADJUST:

>> Your primary goal is fat loss
If after one month your waist circumference is up or unchanged, your progress photos are looking exactly the same, and your weekly bodyweight average is the same or up, this indicates that you have not lost fat. If you've been weight training, it could be possible you have built some muscle. In this case, since your primary goal was to lose fat, an adjustment to caloric intake is required to get fat loss moving at a faster rate. Cutting calories can be accomplished one of two ways:

- Reduce calorie intake by 100-250 calories and recalculate your macros.
- Increasing exercise and/or NEAT levels can achieve the same result as cutting food. If you choose to add cardio, one or two 30-minute low-intensity sessions per week should be sufficient.

On the opposite spectrum, if after a month you are losing weight but constantly tired and fatigued, having trouble sleeping, or lacking energy for your workouts, it's possible your calories are a bit too low. I want this to be a sustainable experience so you can stick with it long-term. You may need to bump up your calorie intake by 100-200 per day, shoot for a high-fiber carbohydrate source to boost energy levels and improve workouts, sleep, and recovery.

>> Your primary goal is muscle gain

After one month, you find that your bodyweight is the same or down, your waist circumference is unchanged or down, and your progress photos appear the same or a bit leaner. It's possible you may have lost fat, but not built much muscle.

Muscle gain can be more difficult to detect than fat loss. If you are gaining strength, it is possible you have built muscle while losing fat. Stick to your plan for another month, keeping track of body part circumference measurements (chest, arms, thighs) to get a better idea of muscle gain. If you have not gained strength, an increase in calories may be beneficial. If you are an advanced lifter, muscle gain is much harder to obtain and detect. Since you likely started with a minimal calorie surplus, an increase in calories may be required for muscle growth at a faster rate.

How many calories you add depends on whether you are losing weight, maintaining weight, or gaining muscle at a slower rate than you'd like. A range of 100-300 additional calories is a good place to start. Remember, building muscle is a SLOW process, so be patient. Rather than constantly switching up your calories and macros, you may also want to take a closer look at your weight training regimen. Muscle growth takes a combination of nutrition and progressive overload to get results. Things like proper form, effort, range of motion, and volume will make or break your results.

Master Your Macros

How Do You Break A Weight-Loss Plateau?

Let's say you've been following your plan for a couple months, and the first 10 pounds seemingly fell off. But then your weekly average weigh-ins go stagnant for four weeks. You're feeling frustrated and ready to give up, so what's next? Plateaus are a normal part of the weight loss journey. The key is working out the reason for the scale halt, so you can adjust accordingly. Go back to Chapter 4 and see how many boxes you can check off the self-assessment in Step 5 of Jumpstart Your Macro Journey." The leaner you get, the more precise and consistent you will need to be with your nutrition to see further results. Here are some reminders of why you are not in a plateau: You struggle with weekends. You have been less than 80-90% consistent with your plan over the last month. It's been less than four weeks of no progress. You stopped tracking calories, getting workouts in, or being as meticulous as you were in the beginning. You aren't looking at your other progress metrics: pics, measurements, body fat%, etc. If you've crossed your t's and dotted your i's, let's get to work on that plateau!

Assess Your Calorie Tracking for Accuracy

Before you make changes, do an honest assessment of your food tracking. An increase in calorie intake so that energy intake matches energy expenditure is the most common reason people hit a weight-loss plateau. Studies have shown it's common to under-report food intake, in some cases by 47% [105]. Some will only track what they want to see while many fail to include bites and nibbles, incorrectly guess portions, take days off, and are simply inconsistent throughout the week.

Adjusting for Metabolic Adaptations of a Plateau

This is an important concept to understand. When someone loses weight, their metabolism decreases no matter what. This isn't a result of metabolic damage, but a natural adaptation. As you lose weight, fewer calories are required by your body to perform the same daily activities. Metabolic adaptations are typically modest at first. As you lose more weight, they may ramp up leading to a much slower rate of weight loss than you might expect. Here's how your metabolism, or "calories out" side of the equation can change as you take in fewer calories and begin to lose weight:

Master Your Macros

- Non-exercise activity thermogenesis (NEAT) decreases. An interesting tip- as you diet longer and get leaner, your body finds subconscious ways to preserve energy, such as less fidgeting and overall body movement. Your NEAT is a large contributor to your overall daily calorie expenditure, and therefore, it accounts for a majority of the metabolic adaptations to dieting. The more moderate your calorie deficit, the less NEAT levels might reduce.
- Thermic Effect of Food (TEF) decreases because you're eating less.
- Basal Metabolic Rate (BMR) decreases because you weigh less. Also, the absence of weight training and sufficient protein intake can result in loss of muscle mass which will slow your metabolism even more.
- Calories burned through physical activity go down simply because you weigh less.

If dietary adherence has been spot on, but neither the scale, nor body measurements have budged in over four weeks, then a true plateau has likely been reached. Plateaus are a normal part of the journey and it means you have successfully reached weight maintenance at a new lower body weight. As your energy balance evolves, so must your strategies for continuing to lose fat. Determining whether you need to decrease calorie intake, increase energy expenditure, do both, or take a diet break will depend on preferences and situation.

HERE ARE SOME GUIDELINES THAT CAN HELP:

- If there is room to decrease calorie intake and hunger levels are not too high, then reducing calories by 100-200 may be the best method.

- If there is room to decrease calorie intake but hunger levels are high, then an increase in activity may be a better option. If calorie intake is already low, then an increase in activity is preferable.

- When increasing activity levels, boosting your NEAT throughout the day may be more beneficial than adding formal cardio since cardio typically results in increased hunger.

- If you find yourself stuck for a few months, it may be time to implement a diet break.

When & How Should You Take a Diet Break?

Diet breaks are a critical component of successful fat loss phases, but people all too commonly skip them. They aren't necessary if you're in a calorie surplus or eating at maintenance, but to be successful with a fat-loss diet, you not only need to know when to make diet adjustments, but also when to take diet breaks. When you have a lot of fat to lose, it can be very tough to stay motivated for months on end, and a diet break will cut up that monotony. When you're trying to reach very low levels of body fat, a diet break helps fight the metabolic adaptations outlined above.

A diet break is exactly what it sounds like: a time of higher calorie intake usually at theoretical maintenance calories (TDEE) for a few days up to a few weeks. Even if you feel like nothing is happening at maintenance, this is where the magic happens for a number of reasons:

- It can be monotonous, and perhaps stressful, to track all the time for some of us. Taking a break and just relaxing once in a while can help mentally. Even knowing the planned break is coming can help you stay on track in between. Vacations are a great time to plan your diet break, as well as relax and enjoy yourself.

- Diet breaks give you more calories, along with more room to fit in the fun stuff! This can mentally help with getting back to dieting when you're ready.

- Some of us experience energy drops and slowdowns when dieting. Consuming more food can boost your NEAT levels and your mood.

- And, one of the lesser talked about benefits is that breaks actually help you practice maintenance. The more practice you have maintaining your weight, the better off you'll be when you hit your final goal.

The goal in including diet breaks is to see your weight loss journey go like this:

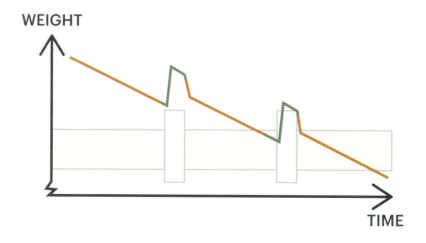

Rather than the diet > binge > quit pattern of many:

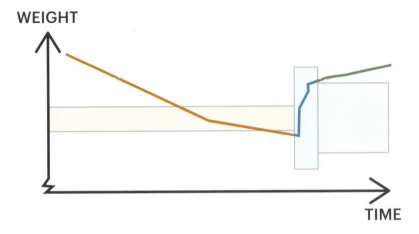

Diet Break Length & Frequency

A diet break can range between a few days to two weeks. The longer you have been dieting, the longer the break may be necessary, since some hormones take longer to recover to normal levels than others. Frequency also depends primarily on our level of leanness. The leaner we get, the more our bodies fight back, so the more frequently diet breaks should be taken:

Body-fat % (Men / Women)	Diet Break Frequency
<10% / 18%	every 6–8 weeks
10-15% / 18–23%	every 8–12 weeks
>15% / >23%	every 12–16 weeks

There are a couple ways to take a diet break

- Stop tracking. Focus on eating to satisfy hunger without overstuffing yourself. Eat at your typical mealtimes, eat slowly, and just enjoy your food until you're satisfied. With these precautions, it's very hard to gain actual fat in a week or two.

- Increase calories to theoretical maintenance (your TDEE) and loosely track. It gives you extra wiggle room to enjoy the foods you love, relaxing your tracking a little but also keeping some constraints for those who like them.

When the diet break is over

- If you were losing weight at your target calorie and macros before the break, return to the same calorie intake after.

- If you were short of your weight loss target, adjust your calorie intake slightly downward. Start with ~100 calories and go from there.

- If the reason you took the diet break was that you were going through a particularly stressful period, and this period coincided with a lower rate of weight loss (or no loss at all), then it's best to assume that water retention was the cause of that. Just return to your previous calorie intake after the break.

How Do You Switch Between Fat Loss & Muscle Gain Goals?

If you've achieved significant progress but remain interested in switching your primary goal, here are some tips that can help the transition:

When to switch from caloric deficit (fat loss) to a caloric surplus (muscle gain)

- Your primary goal has shifted from fat loss to muscle building.
- You have made significant progress and are happy with your current body fat level and overall composition.
- You're extremely lean and it's negatively impacting your health.

When to switch from caloric surplus (muscle gain) to a caloric deficit (fat loss)

- Your primary goal has shifted from building muscle to losing fat.
- You've unintentionally accumulated more body fat than you'd like during your muscle building phase.
- You've been in a surplus for a while and progress has significantly slowed.
- You're feeling tired after your meals and rarely have an appetite.

Set up new calorie and macro calculations based on your new goal. If you have been in a prolonged caloric deficit, you may gradually increase calories over the course of two to three weeks as you transition from deficit to maintenance or surplus, although this is not required. There is no need to gradually transition from a surplus to a deficit.

How Can You Control Hunger?

When dieting, experiencing physical hunger is normal. Increasing our appetite is one of our body's ways of trying to prevent us from losing body mass. By first understanding and accepting that hunger is a normal part of the process, we can save ourselves a little bit of headache. First, it's important to differentiate between emotional and physical hunger.

Emotional Hunger	Physical Hunger
Starts suddenly and feels urgent	Builds gradually over time
Paired with intense emotions	Paired with physical cues (stomach growling, low energy, you're hangry)
Prompts eating past satiety	Dissipates after eating a meal
Accompanied by food fixation	Satisfied by many food options
Often followed by guilt or shame	Not followed by negative emotions

Master Your Macros

During times of heightened stress, it can be hard to tell whether hunger is emotional or physical. Emotional eating is a very common behavior pattern for individuals experiencing high anxiety or charged emotions. It usually starts suddenly in response to a particular trigger or strong emotion and is often accompanied by specific food-fixations or cravings that don't disappear after eating. Those experiencing emotional hunger generally eat far past the point of satiety in an effort to self-soothe.

Physical hunger comes on much slower and is generally paired with physical cues such as a rumbling stomach. You may notice physical hunger because it's been a few hours since your last meal or because your energy levels start to dip. This type of hunger is reduced with a meal or snack, and can be satisfied with any number of food sources. Along with the cues listed above, it's important to note the emotions following physical hunger. If you eat based on physical hunger, your mealtime is not typically followed by negative emotions. In fact, you might not experience any memorable emotions given that eating was not coupled with an emotional trigger. Emotional eating, on the other hand, often comes with guilt or shame, perpetuating negative self-talk.

Changing your behaviors during stressful times, and improving your relationship with food, requires reflection and practice. The first step is becoming conscious of your typical patterns and triggers. If you find that you often turn to food for comfort, understand what cues are influencing the type of hunger you experience so you can navigate them better.

Levels of Physical Hunger & Satiation

I think a lot of us only know two modes of hunger: starving or stuffed. Very rarely do we actually take the time to slow down and understand our physical cues when it comes to hunger. *When we eat, we shouldn't be striving to feel full, but simply to eliminate hunger.* The hunger scale is a great way to articulate this sometimes vague sensation accompanying varying degrees of physical hunger.

1-2 on a regular basis might be improved with better meal timing, better food choices, or more calories.

Fat loss is usually at a 3-5 or below

Weight maintenance is a 6 or below

6 and above on a regular basis and you're typically in muscle building or fat gain territory.

1. Starving and feeling weak/dizzy
2. Very hungry; cranky; low energy; hunger pangs
3. Pretty hungry; stomach growling a little
4. Starting to feel a little hungry
5. Satisfied; neither hungry nor full
6. A little full/pleasantly full
7. Slightly full; a little uncomfortable
8. Feeling stuffed; heaviness in stomach
9. Very uncomfortable; stomach hurts
10. So full you feel sick

Make Strategic Food Choices

Satiety, or fullness, can make all the difference on your fat loss journey. A study on the "Satiety Index" compared how filling 240 calories is among various foods- white bread was the baseline at 100%. Hunger was measured every 15 minutes and participants were free to eat over the following 2 hours. The top satiety food performers: Potatoes 323%, Ling Fish 225%, Oatmeal 209%, Oranges 202%, Apples 197%, Brown Pasta 188%, Beef 176%, Baked Beans 168%, Popcorn 154% and Eggs 150% [182].

Fatty foods by themselves, contrary to what most people think, are not filling. Essentially, the more protein, fiber and volume the food provides in relation to its calorie content, the more filling it is. These foods literally fill your stomach and digest slowly, so you feel fuller longer. Makes sense based on what you've learned in this guide, right?

While it's totally fine to fit some of your favorite indulgences into your diet, prioritizing lean protein and fibrous veggies at a majority of your meals will help you combat normal feelings of hunger. *Why not give a few of my high-protein recipes in Chapter 11 a try!*

Understand Exercise's Impact on Hunger Levels

High intensity cardio in particular can often leave us feeling hungrier and/or tired over the remainder of the day, so plan around this by either scaling back on the frequency and/or intensity or plan your meals around your cardio.

Distract Yourself

Hunger might feel like the worst thing in the world if you allow yourself to STEW in it. Get up and do something else! You might be surprised at how effective distraction is. Because if you get moving by tidying up or cleaning, you can also boost your NEAT, and enjoy a clean house!

What Else Can You Do to Improve Your Progress?

When it comes to fat loss and muscle gain, training and nutrition are two variables that work hand-in-hand. However, there are other life variables you can control to make the journey even more successful.

Weight Train Regularly

We know strength training builds muscle, but it's also one of the most misunderstood fat loss tools. A regular strength training regimen is critical in every goal for a few reasons:

> Muscle mass is a large part of your metabolism—the more muscle mass you have, the more calories you burn at rest. If you need a refresher on the importance of muscle for your metabolism, especially with retention as we age, see Chapter 1.

> Strength training offsets the likelihood of muscle catabolism that caloric restriction induces. In fact, for every pound lost through diet, up to 25% can come from muscle tissue [183–185]. And the larger the percentage of weight loss from muscle mass during a diet the bigger likelihood of subsequent weight regain [186]. To help preserve metabolic muscle tissue, resistance training in combination with a high protein diet tells your body to burn fat and preserve and/or build as much muscle as possible.

> Due to increased post exercise oxygen consumption, weight training causes your body to burn calories during and long after your session. Whereas with cardio, you essentially stop burning calories when your session ends. According to a recent study, just ten weeks of weight training could boost calories burned at rest by 7% and may reduce fat by four pounds [183, 184].

De-Stress

Feeling strung out? Anxiety out of control? To be healthy, you simply have to get a hold of your stress levels, especially if you're a high stress person. If your fitness program makes you stressed, find a different program that works better for you. If you're stressed outside the fitness world (work, home, life, etc.), finding ways to cope with that is important. Stress makes losing weight a lot harder and less fun. It can mess with hormones too, which is why many people eat when they become stressed. To add insult to injury, a rise in cortisol from the stress can cause our bodies to hold more water, making us feel "softer" and "less lean" than we actually are. If you're stressed, talk to someone you trust. Take walks. Some find that meditation and yoga really do the trick.

Balance Your Hormones

As we covered in Chapter 1, hormones and metabolism are intertwined. As we covered in Chapter 2, many of the foods we eat impact the hormones that control hunger, fullness, and how our body burns and stores calories. There are many other hormone factors to consider too. The thyroid changes how many calories our body burns. Hypothyroidism results in fewer calories burned, whereas Hyperthyroidism will burn slightly more calories. Women experiencing menopause will experience elevated Follicle-stimulating hormones (FSH) and suppress estrogen. Having low testosterone, high testosterone, or low estrogen levels can change how quickly you put on muscle and how hard it is to lose fat. Polycystic Ovary Syndrome (PCOS), a hormonal disorder common among women of reproductive age, typically results in high testosterone levels, low progesterone levels, and reduced insulin sensitivity. Any hormone imbalance can make both fat loss and muscle gain extremely challenging. If you suspect any hormone imbalances, seek medical attention for appropriate corrective measures.

Get Enough Sleep

If you recall from Chapter 7, quality sleep plays an important role in weight management, health, and well-being. Without sufficient sleep, both muscle building and fat loss can be hard. Sleep deprivation is associated with an increase in obesity among men by 3.7 times, and a 2.3-fold increase in obesity among women, compared to those who sleep seven to eight hours per night [145]. Essentially, when we don't get enough sleep, our bodies want/need more energy. As a result, it produces more ghrelin (the hormone that makes us hungry) and decreases leptin (the hormone that helps us feel full). A systematic review of eleven studies concluded poor sleep patterns resulted in an average of 385 extra calories consumed per day [123]! So, don't just aim for six to eight hours, aim for six to eight *quality hours*.

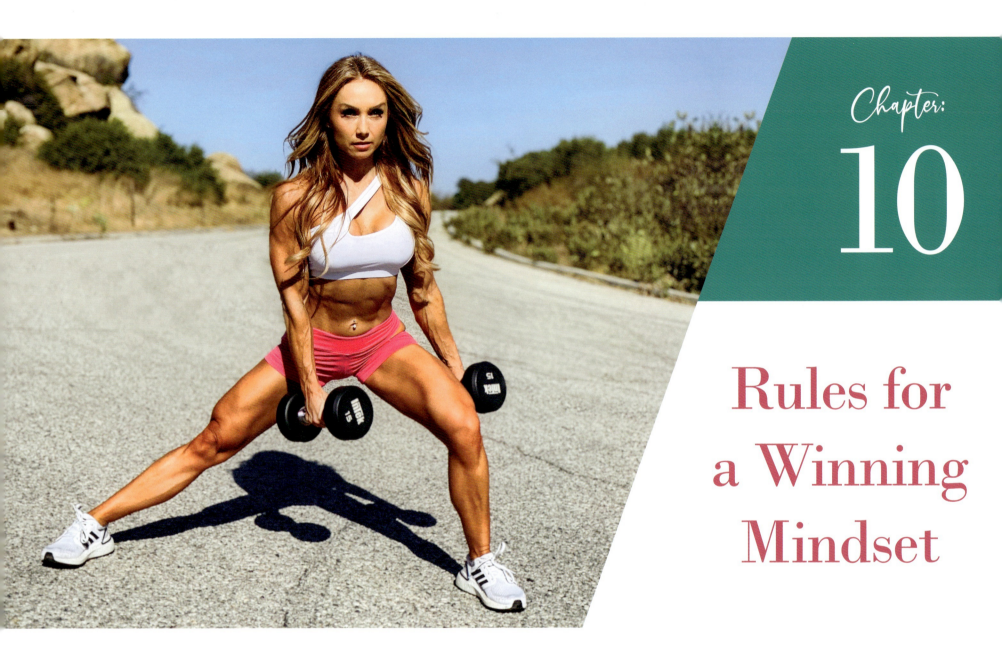

Chapter: 10

Rules for a Winning Mindset

I know it can be so exciting to start a new plan, and you might want to go all in within the first week.
While enthusiasm is a good thing, you don't want to set too many goals then feel disappointed when they aren't met. The truth is we are all creatures of habit. It has taken us years of various life circumstances to build these habits, and some might be standing in the way of reaching our goals, such as: your upbringing, work, kids, culture, community, and values. Some habits are deeply rooted and harder to break than others. It's unrealistic to expect to wake up tomorrow, completely overhaul your approach to nutrition, and never face setbacks, roadblocks, or feel a little struggle.

Replacing old, bad eating habits with new, healthier ones is not an easy task. You are building a new you. Practice, experience, and patience are the foundation of change. Now that you have knowledge on how to use nutrition to increase your energy, lose fat, and build muscle, how you go about it will determine your long-term success. If you want to get and stay lean and strong, you have to embrace a new lifestyle full of habits that support a lean, strong and healthy body.

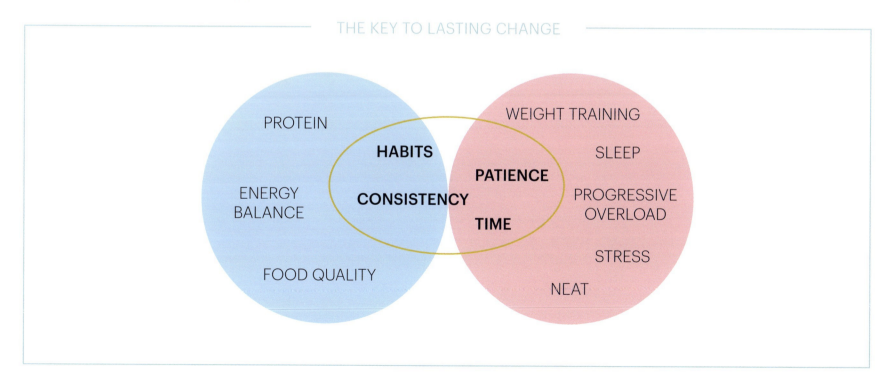

THE KEY TO LASTING CHANGE

Master Your Macros

01 Consistency, Not Perfection

Without consistency, you will never achieve your goals, plain and simple. But there's a big difference between being consistent and seeking perfection. As it turns out, the all-or-nothing mentality, black-and-white, or dichotomous thinking in the scientific literature, is considered a form of cognitive, or mental rigidity that ultimately does more harm than good. There are ways that this mindset can hold you back as it relates to fitness and health.

You may be more likely to:
- See yourself as either a "success" or "failure"
- Categorize foods as good/bad, healthy/unhealthy
- Starve then overeat / binge-eat
- Continue to yo-yo diet
- Have lower well-being and higher body dissatisfaction

Every single one of us deviates from our nutrition and exercise plan from time to time, whether it's unplanned snacks or one-pound burgers, extra fries, and a 20 ounce shake. We're not robots, we're human. Our behavior is more complex than simply "doing the thing and making no mistakes." Plus, there's a whole middle ground that gets completely overlooked when the only options are 0 or 100. More often than not, I'd argue that all-or-nothing leaves you with, well, nothing. It's those who focus on consistently doing their best, learning from mistakes, and getting back to consistency that always win. Essentially, what separates those who succeed from those who fail is how they respond to the screw ups.

From now on, I want you to embrace the fact that mistakes happen. Learn from them, grow from them, and never let a few mistakes keep you from getting back on track.

02 Restraint As Opposed To Restriction

To get lean and strong, you will likely have to eat fewer calories, eat more protein, and consume less junk food. It's not that you can't have the more indulgent foods, but you choose to limit them for a greater goal.

You are the one in control of your diet and exercise choices. Your fitness plan doesn't control you. More often than not, restriction, or "good" vs. "bad" food labeling, leads to a worse relationship with food, more cravings, resentment towards your nutrition plan, and eventually binges. On the other hand, restraint creates empowerment and ownership over your food choices. When you feel empowered to make good food choices, you ultimately end up "restraining" from the ones that are keeping you from getting to your goals without even thinking about it.

Be empowered knowing that you are 100% in control. That ownership might scare you now, but in time, it will empower you! Of course, it can be difficult to restrain yourself from eating the entire box of Oreos or a whole pizza in the moment, but that difficulty gets shadowed by the happiness that comes from reaching your goals and feeling in control of your choices.

03 Something Small Versus Nothing

Reading this guide is one small step in the right direction. You now know how much and what foods best support your goals. Why not take that same one-step-at-a-time approach to your goals? If you struggle to control every meal in your day, how about just one or two of them? **Each meal, snack, and small step in the right direction is better than none at all.**

Remember: consistency with the meals you can control is always better than changing nothing. Because every improvement, no matter how small, adds up to long lasting results. I suggest setting one to two realistic goals every week and/or month that supports your big picture. Write it down and identify what it will take each day to work towards this goal, then hold yourself accountable.

For example, if your goal is to stick to the calorie budget you calculated, what changes do you need to make for this to happen? Maybe this is practicing logging foods in *Lose It!* and trying out a few recipes in this guide. Other great weekly goals might include:

- Eat a serving of lean protein with each meal.
- Fill half your plate with colorful fruits and vegetables.
- Substitute saturated or trans fats for unsaturated fats.
- Switch to primarily calorie-free drinks.
- Eat more slowly – put the fork down in between bites. Focus on the food: its taste, texture, and smells.
- Eat until you're a 4 or 5 on the hunger scale (see Chapter 9). Once you are about a 4 stop your meal and allow your body time to adjust to feeling satiated.

Non-food related goals might include:
- Drink eight glasses of water to stay hydrated throughout the day.
- Set a new sleeping schedule, aim for seven to eight hours each night.
- Take a five-minute walking break to avoid sitting for more than three hours at a time.
- Celebrate your wins and revisit any of these habits you are still having trouble maintaining.

Instead of feeling like you have to completely overhaul your nutrition plan, making small tweaks every week may be the best option to avoid feeling deprived.

	Current Eating Habits	New, Small Changes
7am:	Veggie omelet with cheese, hash browns, toast and butter	Veggie omelet with avocado and a Pumpkin Oatmeal muffin
10am	Bag of Doritos	Tuna with crackers
12pm	Hamburger, fries and regular soda	Hamburger, apple and diet soda
3pm:	Granola bar	Birthday Cake Protein Bar
7pm:	Chicken tacos with chips and salsa	Chicken tacos with side of broccoli

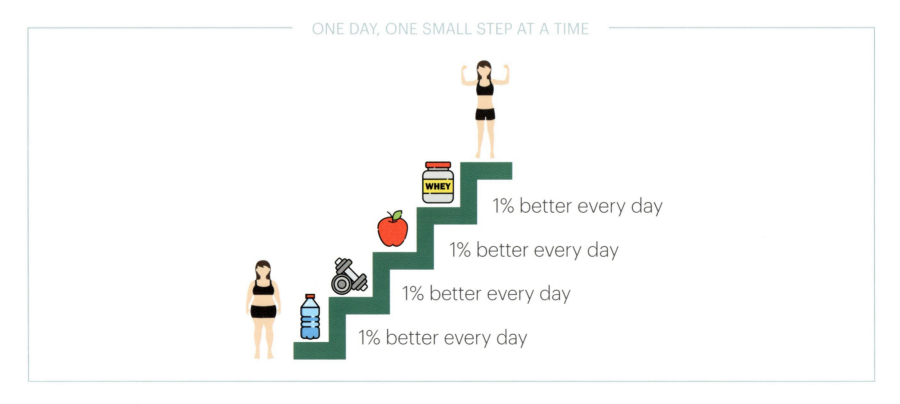

ONE DAY, ONE SMALL STEP AT A TIME

1% better every day
1% better every day
1% better every day
1% better every day

Master Your Macros

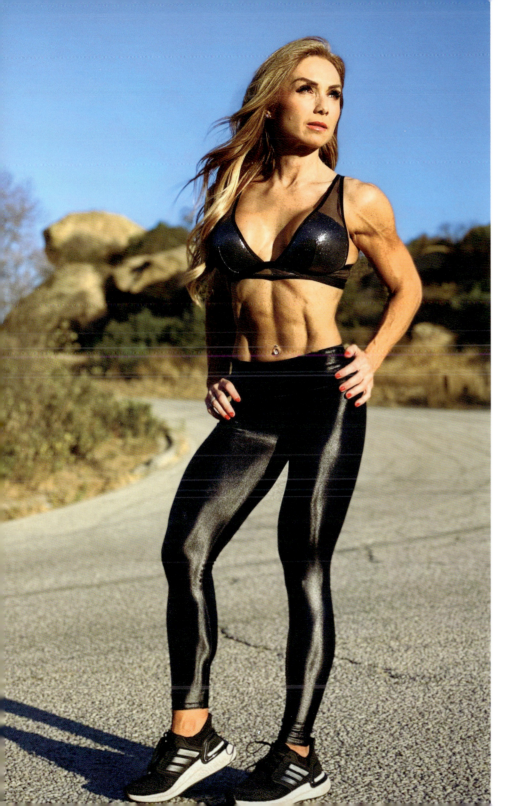

"Be Stubborn About Your Goals and Flexible About Your Methods."

-Unknown

I love this quote! It could apply to just about anything, couldn't it? You want to raise good kids. You want the dog not to pee inside the house. You want a fantastic relationship with your significant other that is full of love and respect. Some goals are easier said than done, and navigating your nutrition is no exception.

I hope this guide has helped you understand that just because a nutrition plan didn't work in the past doesn't mean you need to give up on your health and fitness goals. You likely only required a different method. One that helps you get to know yourself better, teaches you what it takes to reach your goals (not just tell you what to do), keeps you motivated and consistent. And I wholeheartedly believe the information and tips I've provided in this guide will help you with all of these!

Stay focused, be flexible, show up every day to the behaviors of the person you want to become, and I promise this will all become automatic in no time. You can always come back here for some guidance along the way.

I know you are ready to Master Your Macros!

Success Story

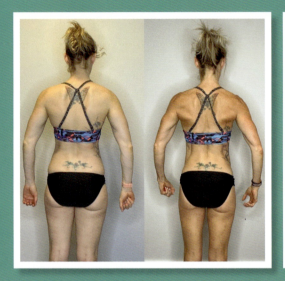
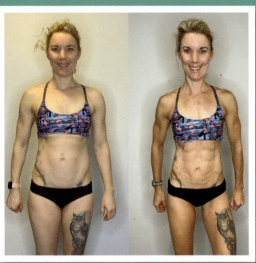

"In just four months I lost 10 pounds and regained control over my nutrition"

I'm not your typical transformation story. I struggled for many years with an eating disorder, was underweight, headed down a dark path of food restriction, binging, and purging. I was forced to face the consequences of my unhealthy lifestyle in 2008 when my family threatened to take my son away. It was the wakeup call I couldn't be more thankful for.

Over the last four years, I really dove into my own health, and discovered a newfound love for fitness while helping others. Then March 2020 came, and, like many others, COVID-19 turned my world upside down. The stress of homeschooling my children, working from home, and finishing my Master's degree was copied through comfort foods like candy, chips, and ice cream. The "Quarantine 15" became my new reality.

While unhappy that I let my healthy habits slip, this was a much smaller hurdle than I've faced in the past. My mind became fixed on bigger goals to build a lean, strong physique, and there's was no better time than this moment to tackle it. I wanted, however, to be sure I went about it the right way. I did some research, and when I came across Breanne's macro-based nutrition approach to blast fat and build muscle is when everything changed. I began with a fat loss goal, calculated my calories and macros, downloaded the *Lose It!* app. With Breanne's simple tips and guidance, I gave the plan everything I had.

> *In just four months I lost 10 pounds and regained control over my nutrition. I see changes in my body that I've never seen before—things that I love! At 39, I'm healthier, leaner, running faster, and stronger mentally, physically, and emotionally.*

Through this process I've learned so much about the foods I eat. Focusing on appropriate levels of protein, carbs and fat has made the biggest impact on my results. It has reduced the cravings for comfort foods, and I now see this exactly what my body needs for proper recovery after a heavy lift or a long run. With the data right at my fingertips, I can also fit treats I want without guilt– something I never could have imagined feeling before. This is no longer a "diet," but a lifestyle that both my husband and I love. I'm so excited with these results, I'm considering a bikini competition for my 40th birthday. Thanks Breanne!

- Maygan Lenz

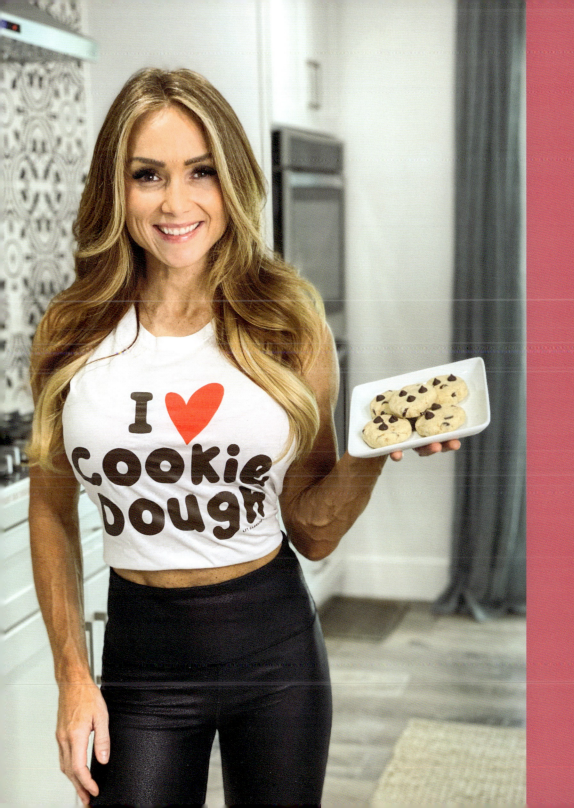

Recipes That Fit Your *Macros*

....

GETTING LEAN AND STRONG HAS NEVER TASTED SO GOOD!

I've taken your favorite foods - like pizza, burgers, pasta, cakes, cookies, cheesecake, ice cream, and brownies - and made them high-protein, low-calorie, and super tasty! I want to show you can have fun with your food, actually enjoy what you eat, and still reach your goals.

Things to Know

Navigation:
If you're reading the digital e-book version, you can click on any recipe title on the next page and jump straight to the recipe.

Calorie and Macro Calculations
You'll find a full macro breakdown of every recipe at the bottom of every page: Cal= Calories, F=Fat, C=Carbs, P= Protein. Calculations are the based on the specific brands, ingredients, and specified serving sizes. Macros may vary per brand and product, so I recommend using the Lose It! app recipes feature (see Chapter 6) to determine the calories and macros of any recipe you make. A shopping list of many of my recipe ingredients is available at www.amazon.com/shop/breannefreeman

Recipe Substitutions
Use different ingredients or change the serving size of any recipe to fit your preference, calorie, and macro requirements. Please note I haven't tested the recipes with any other ingredients other than those specified. Using a different protein powder is inherently risky. If at all possible, use a similar whey/casein blend, or match gram for gram, and not scoop for scoop. Vegan proteins tend to be very thick and require additional moisture, and whey protein isolates can end up dry in baked goods and runny when mixed in foods like oatmeal. While the recipes are not vegan/plant-based, you're free to give them a try with any plant-based substitutions:

Whey Protein → Soy, Hemp, Pea Protein Powder

Greek Yogurt → Almond, Coconut or Soy Yogurt, Vegan Sour Cream

Cheese → Vegan Cheddar or Mozzarella Style Shreds, Vegan Parmesan, Vegan Cream Cheese, Vegan Ricotta, Vegan Cheese Slices

Meats → Plant-Based Crumbles, Coconut or Tempeh Bacon Pulled Jackfruit, Seitan, Tempeh, Textured Vegetable Protein, Tofu (Plain or Flavored), Vegan Burgers, Vegan Chicken or Beef Strips, Vegan Deli Slices, Vegan Meatballs, Nuggets, and Sausages

Recipes

Breakfasts

Blackberry Ricotta Protein Pancakes.............144
Strawberry Protein Shortcakes......................145
Cocoa Mocha Protein Bowl............................146
Almond Joy Overnight Oats............................147
Banana Bread Protein Oats.............................148
Chocolate Peanut Butter Protein Bake..........149
Berry Breakfast Protein Pizza........................150
Cinnamon Roll Protein French Toast............151
Deep Dish Breakfast Pizza..............................152
Breakfast Egg Muffins....................................153
Loaded Breakfast Quesadilla.........................154
Egg & Bacon Cream Cheese Bagels..............155

Breads

Rainbow Sprinkle Protein Donuts..................156
Double Chocolate Protein Donuts.................157
Blueberry Lemon Protein Muffins.................158
Pumpkin Pecan Oat Protein Muffins.............159
Banana Chocolate Chip Protein Bread.........160
Chocolate Strawberry Protein Bread............161
Everything Protein Bagels..............................162
Rosemary Focaccia Protein Bread.................163

Main Dishes

Egg Salad Slimwich..164
Apple Walnut Tuna Salad Wrap.....................165
Chicken, Bacon Ranch Street Tacos..............166
Cheesy Chicken & Cauliflower Rice..............167
Pepperoni Protein Pizza..................................168
Turkey Bacon Cheeseburger Flatbread.........169
Turkey Enchiladas...170
Greek Meatball Wrap w/ Tzatziki
     Herb Yogurt Sauce....................................171
Turkey Sloppy (Thin) Joes..............................172
Taco Fiesta Bites..173
Beef Nacho Salad...174
Cheesy Beef & Spinach Lasagna Cups..........175
Spicy Beef Mac & Cheese...............................176
Blackbean Quesadilla Burgers.......................177
Avocado Cilantro Salmon Meatballs &
     Zucchini Spaghetti....................................178
Protein Corn Dogs w/ Maple
     Dijon Mustard..179

Desserts

Chocolate Chip Protein Cookies....................180
Fudge Protein Brownies.................................181
Chocolate Peanut Butter Protein Eggs.........182
Vanilla Raspberry Protein Mini Cheesecake....183
Chocolate & Vanilla Swirl Protein Cupcakes....184
Funfetti Protein Cake......................................185
Rocky Road Protein Ice Cream......................186
Chocolate Chip Protein Cookie Dough.........187
Protein Brownie Batter...................................188

Snacks

Birthday Cake Protein Bars............................189
Strawberry Cheesecake
     Protein Parfait...190
Blueberry Muffin Protein Pudding................191
Banana Almond Protein Dip..........................192
Spicy Avocado Protein Toast.........................193
Soft Protein Pretzels with Nacho
     Cheese Dip...194
Margherita Pizza Protein Pocket..................195

Master Your Macros

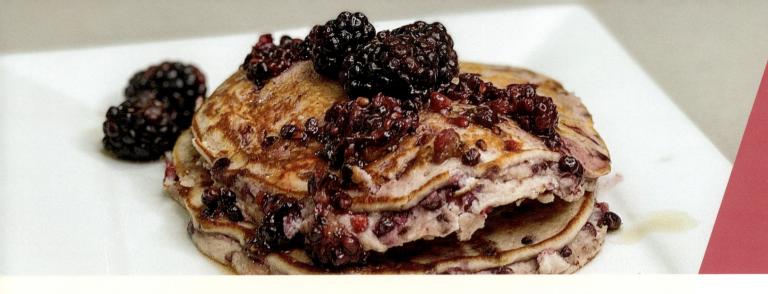

Breakfasts

Blackberry Ricotta Protein Pancakes

1. Spray your griddle with non-stick cooking spray and preheat over low heat.
2. Mash black berries in a bowl.
3. In a separate bowl whisk egg and ricotta until smooth.
4. Add whey protein, coconut flour and cinnamon. Mix well.
5. Fold in mashed blackberries.
6. When the griddle is hot, pour 1/4 of the batter per pancake. Flip when you see the bottom of the pancake browning.
7. Cook for 1-2 more minutes. Repeat until you've finished your batter.
8. Top 2 pancakes with 4 tbsp sugar-free maple syrup. Enjoy!

Ingredients:
+ 1/2 cup (120g) liquid egg whites
+ 1/2 cup (124g) low fat ricotta
+ 46g (1.5 scoops) Quest Vanilla Milkshake protein powder
+ 1 tbsp (7g) coconut flour
+ 1 cup (144g) blackberries, mashed
+ Dash of cinnamon
+ 1/2 cup (120mL) sugar-free maple syrup

Makes 2 servings, 2 pancakes each:
Cal: 233, F: 2.7g, C: 23.5g (5g fiber), P: 31g

Enjoy in 15 minutes
⏰ Prep time: **10**   🍲 Cook time: **5**

Master Your Macros

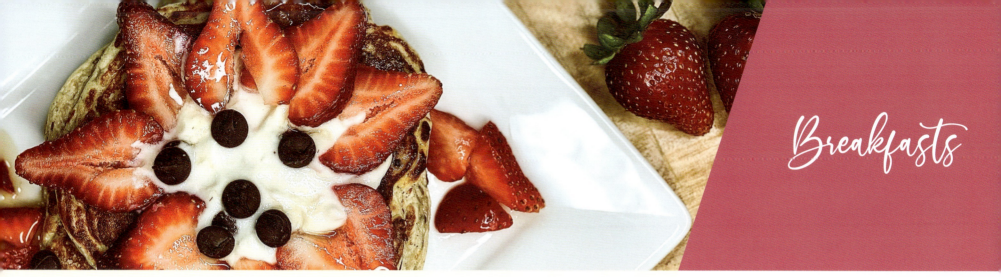

Breakfasts

Strawberry Protein Shortcakes

1. Beat egg whites, Greek yogurt and vanilla extract until smooth.
2. Mix in protein powder, oats, coconut flour and baking powder.
3. Fold in 1/2 cup diced strawberries. The batter will thicken as it sits for a few minutes.
4. Spray your griddle with non-stick cooking spray and heat to medium. When hot, add around 1/4 cup of the batter for each pancake. Flip after 1-2 minutes or when the bottom of the pancake is brown. Cook for 1-2 more minutes. Repeat until you've finished your batter.
5. Top two pancakes with 1/5 vanilla protein frosting, diced strawberries and syrup (chocolate chips optional). Enjoy!

Pancake Ingredients:
+ 62g (2 scoops) Quest Vanilla Milkshake protein powder
+ 1 1/3 cup (320g) liquid egg whites
+ 1/2 cup (40g) quick oats
+ 2/3 cup (160g) 0% plain Greek yogurt
+ 4 tbsp (28g) coconut flour
+ 2 tsp (8g) baking powder
+ 1 tsp (4g) vanilla extract
+ 1 1/2 cups (300g) strawberries, diced
+ 1/2 cup (120mL) sugar-free maple syrup

Vanilla Protein Frosting:
+ 31g (1 scoop) Quest Vanilla Milkshake protein powder
+ 1/2 cup (120g) 0% plain Greek yogurt

Makes 5 servings, 2 pancakes each:
Cal: 210, F: 1.5g, C: 21.5g (4.4g fiber), P: 27.5g

Enjoy in 20 minutes
Prep time: 10   Cook time: 10

Master Your Macros

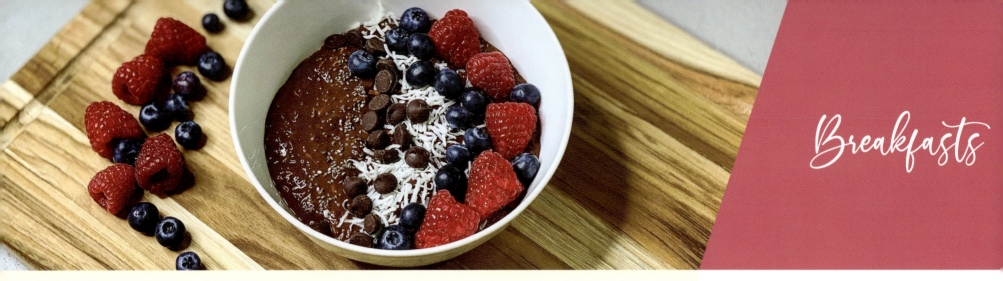

Breakfasts

Cocoa Mocha Protein Bowl

1. Mix protein powder, coffee, milk, chia seeds, coconut, vanilla extract and cocoa powder in a bowl.
2. Cover and refrigerate for at least 2 hours to allow chia seeds to absorb moisture.
3. Top with berries and chocolate chips and enjoy.

Ingredients:
- 31g (1 scoop) Quest Chocolate Milkshake protein powder
- 3/4 cup (180mL) unsweetened cashew/almond milk
- 2 tbsp (26g) chia seeds
- 2 tbsp (10g) unsweetened shredded coconut
- 1 tbsp (5g) cocoa powder
- 2 tsp (4g) espresso instant coffee
- 1 tsp (4g) vanilla extract
- 1 1/2 tbsp (14g) Lily's chocolate chips
- 1/4 cup (25g) blueberries
- 1/4 cup (30g) raspberries

Makes 1 serving:
Cal: 422 , F: 19.5g, C: 34g (21g fiber), P: 30g

Enjoy in 125 minutes
Prep time: **5**   Cook time: **2 hours**

Master Your Macros

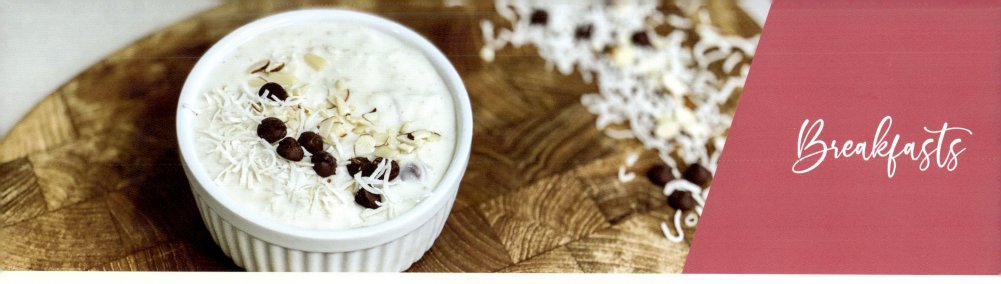

Almond Joy Overnight Oats

1. Mix ingredients in a bowl and let it sit overnight in your refrigerator. Enjoy cold!

Ingredients:

+ 1/4 cup (20g) quick oats
+ 1 scoop (31g) Quest Vanilla Milkshake Protein Powder
+ 1/2 cup (120mL) unsweetened cashew/almond or cashew milk
+ 1/2 cup (120g) Light & Fit Vanilla Greek yogurt
+ 2 tbsp (14g) Lily's chocolate chips
+ 1 tbsp (5g) shredded unsweetened coconut
+ 1 tbsp (5g) sliced almonds
+ 1/2 tsp (2g) coconut extract

Makes 1 serving:
Cal: 400, F: 13.5g, C: 37g (8g fiber), P: 42g

Enjoy in 12 hours 5 minutes
Prep time: **5** / Let sit for **12** hours

Master Your Macros

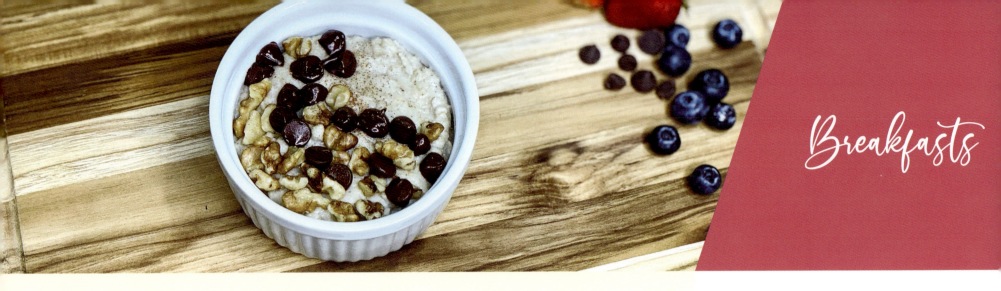

Banana Bread Protein Oats

Ingredients:

+ 31g (1 scoop) Quest Vanilla Milkshake protein powder
+ 1/4 cup (20g) quick oats
+ 1/2 cup (120g) water
+ 1/2 overripe small banana (50g), mashed
+ 1/4 tsp (1g) vanilla extract
+ 1/4 tsp (1g) butter extract
+ 1 tbsp (10g) Lily's chocolate chips
+ 1 tbsp (7g) chopped walnuts
+ Cinnamon to taste

1. In a microwave-safe bowl, combine the oats, mashed banana and water. Microwave for one minute.
2. Remove oats from the microwave and stir in the protein powder, vanilla extract, butter extract and cinnamon. Add additional water if needed for desired consistency.
3. Top with walnuts, chocolate chips and enjoy!

Additional optional toppings: blueberries, strawberries, sliced bananas.

Makes 1 serving:
Cal: 320, F: 10.5g, C: 34.5g (6g fiber), P: 29g

Enjoy in 7 minutes
Prep time: **6**   Cook time: **1**

Master Your Macros

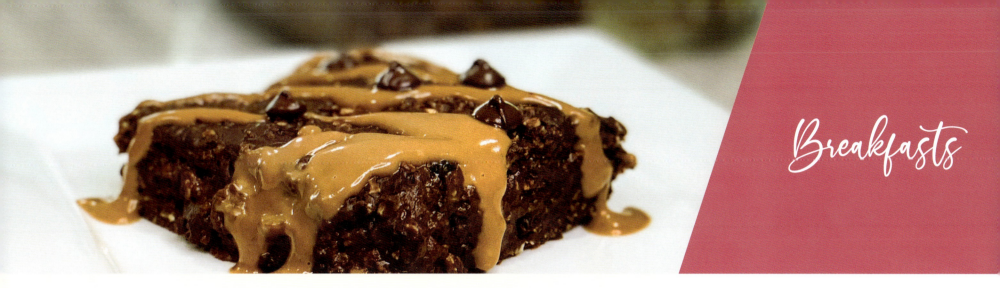

Chocolate Peanut Butter Cup Breakfast Bake

1. Preheat oven to 350°F and spray 8"x8" baking dish with non-stick spray.
2. Mix the dry ingredients in a large bowl.
3. Add the pumpkin, applesauce, peanut butter and milk. Mix well, it will be thick.
4. Transfer to your baking dish, smooth the top of the mixture, top with chocolate chips and bake for 12-18 minutes (depending on how soft you like it).
5. Mix peanut butter drizzle ingredients.
6. Cut the breakfast bake into 4 slices, top with 1/4 the peanut butter drizzle. Enjoy!

Ingredients:
- 1 cup (80g) quick oats
- 90g (3 scoops) Quest Chocolate Milkshake Protein Powder
- 1/4 cup (20g) unsweetened cocoa powder
- 3 tbsp (18g) powdered peanut butter
- 1/2 cup (120g) unsweetened applesauce
- 2/3 cup (160mL) unsweetened cashew/almond milk
- 1/2 cup (120g) canned pumpkin
- 1 tbsp (14g) Breanne's Blend Cookie Batter peanut butter
- 1/2 tsp (2g) baking powder
- 2 tbsp (21g) Lily's semi-sweet chocolate chips

Peanut Butter Drizzle:
- 4 tbsp (24g) powdered peanut butter
- 2 tbsp (30mL) unsweetened cashew milk
- 2 tsp (6g) Swerve confectioners' sugar substitute

Makes 4 servings, each:
Cal: 275, F: 6.5g, C: 35g (9g fiber), P: 28g

Enjoy in 25 minutes
Prep time: **10**   Cook time: **15**

Master Your Macros

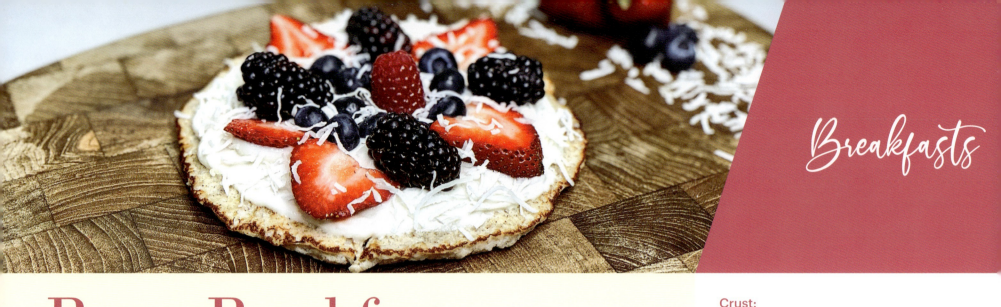

Berry Breakfast Protein Pizza

1. Add crust ingredients into a bowl and whisk together until smooth.
2. Preheat the griddle to medium heat. Spray with non-stick spray and add half the crust batter.
3. Spread the batter around in the pan to flatten the batter and form the circular shape of your crust. Add a cover to the pan and cook for 1-2 minutes.
4. Spray the top of the crust with nonstick cooking spray and flip it over. Press edges down with the spatula to prevent curling. Cook on that side for another 1-2 minutes or until browned. Repeat this process with the second half of your batter.
5. Mix frosting ingredients in a small bowl.
6. Top cooked crusts with 1/2 frosting, berries, shredded coconut and enjoy!

Makes 2 breakfast pizzas, each:
Cal: 263, F:3.5g, C: 32g (9.5g fiber), P: 23g

Enjoy in 25 minutes
Prep time: **15**   Cook time: **10**

Crust:
+ 1 overripe small banana (100g), mashed
+ 3/4 cup (180g) liquid egg whites
+ 4 tbsp (14g) coconut flour
+ 2 tbsp (30mL) sugar-free maple syrup
+ 1/2 tsp (2g) vanilla extract
+ 1/2 tsp (2g) cinnamon

Frosting:
+ 1/3 cup (80g) 0% plain Greek yogurt
+ 1/2 scoop (15g) Quest Vanilla Milkshake protein powder
+ 1/4 cup (60mL) sugar-free maple syrup
+ 1/2 tsp (2g) vanilla extract

Toppings:
+ 100g mixed berries: blueberries, strawberries, blackberries, raspberries
+ 1 tbsp (10g) unsweetened shredded coconut

Breakfasts

Master Your Macros

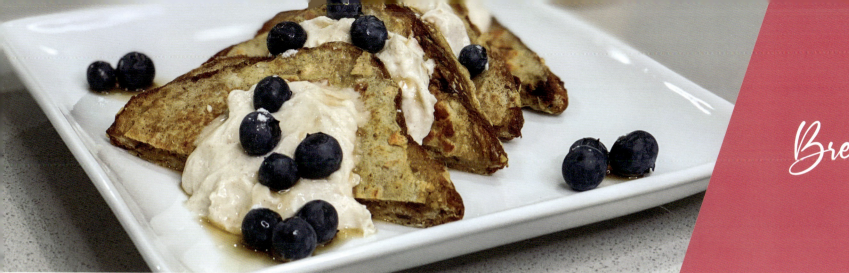

Cinnamon Roll Protein French Toast

1. Preheat griddle to medium heat.
2. In a large baking dish, whisk 1 scoop protein powder, eggs, almond milk, vanilla extract, cinnamon and salt.
3. Mix frosting ingredients in a separate bowl.
4. Cut each slice of bread diagonally to make 8 triangles. Soak each slice in the egg mixture for about 1 minute per side.
5. Spray griddle with non-stick spray and cook bread for 1-2 minutes per side, or until golden brown.
6. Top each piece with 1/8 frosting mix and enjoy. Optional toppings: berries, Lily's chocolate chips, sugar-free maple syrup.

Ingredients:
- 4 slices Raisin' The Roof Dave's Killer Bread
- 31g (1 scoop) Quest Cinnamon Crunch protein powder
- 2 large eggs (100g)
- 1/4 cup (60mL) unsweetened cashew/almond milk
- 1/2 tsp (2g) vanilla extract
- 1/2 tsp (1g) cinnamon
- Pinch of salt

Cinnamon Roll Protein Frosting:
- 31g (1 scoop) Quest Cinnamon Crunch protein powder
- 1/2 cup (120g) 0% plain Greek yogurt
- 2 tbsp (30mL) sugar-free maple syrup
- Dash of cinnamon

Makes 2 servings, each:
Cal: 410, F: 8g, C: 44g (4.5g fiber), P: 38g

Enjoy in 20 minutes
Prep time: 10   Cook time: 10

Master Your Macros

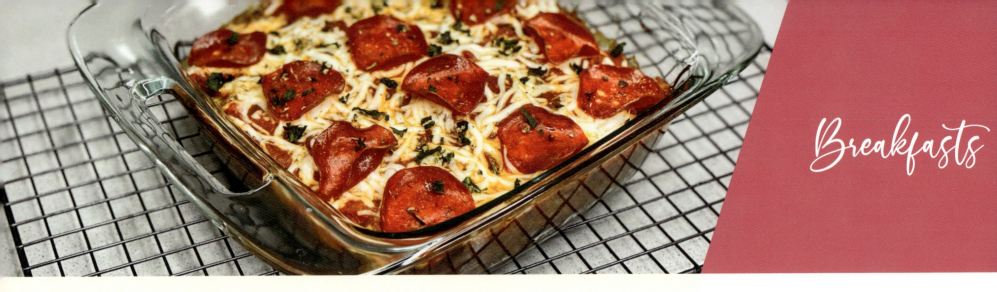

Deep Dish Breakfast Pizza

1. Preheat your oven to 450°F. Cook frozen veggies in a stove top pan over medium heat with cover on until they start to soften. Add salt and mix until they begin to char.
2. Spray an 8"x8" baking dish with non-stick cooking spray and distribute cooked veggies along the bottom.
3. In a bowl whisk together eggs, egg whites, ricotta cheese, coconut flour, oregano, basil, and garlic powder. Pour mixture evenly on top veggies in your baking dish.
4. Bake for 25 minutes, then add marinara, mozzarella, Turkey pepperoni, and return to the oven for another 8-10 minutes.
5. Once cooked, sprinkle a little more oregano, garlic and basil top to taste. Slice and enjoy!

Ingredients:
- (2) 12oz. bags (680g) frozen broccoli & cauliflower
- 1/2 cup (120g) liquid egg whites
- 2 large eggs (100g)
- 1/4 cup (60g) part skim ricotta cheese
- 2 tbsp (24g) coconut flour
- 3/4 cup (183g) marinara sauce
- 1/2 cup (56g) reduced-fat shredded mozzarella cheese
- 12 slices (21g) reduced-fat turkey pepperoni
- 1 tsp (1g) oregano
- 1 tsp (1g) garlic powder
- 1 tsp (1g) dried basil
- 1-2 tsp salt

Makes 4 slices, each:
Cal: 250, F: 9g, C: 19g (6.5g fiber), P: 23.5g

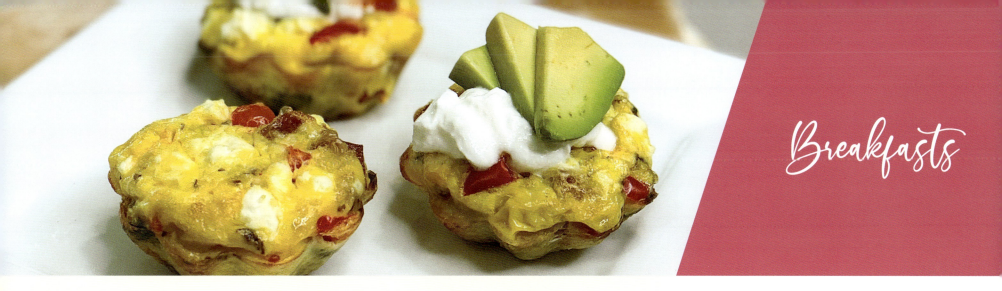

Breakfast Egg Muffins

1. Preheat oven to 350°F, coat 12-cup muffin tin with non-stick spray.
2. Divide spinach, red bell pepper, tomatoes among the cups until they are about 2/3 full.
3. In a large bowl whisk together the eggs, salt, basil, oregano, and pepper.
4. Divide egg mixture between each cup and top with 1 tsp feta cheese each.
5. Bake for 25 minutes. Let cool for a few minutes, then run a knife around the edges of each muffin to loosen it. Remove muffins from the pan, add additional toppings and enjoy!

Optional toppings: avocado, salsa, hot sauce, 0% plain Greek yogurt, freshly chopped parsley.

Ingredients:
- 6 large eggs (300g)
- 3/4 cup (180g) liquid egg whites
- 4 slices Godshalls Fully Cooked Uncured Turkey Bacon, diced
- 1 cup (225g) baby spinach, chopped
- 1/2 cup (90g) red bell pepper, finely diced
- 3/4 cup (150g) quartered cherry tomatoes
- 1/4 tsp (1g) sea salt
- 1/4 tsp (0.2g) dried basil
- 1/4 tsp (0.2g) dried oregano
- 1oz. (28g) fat-free crumbled feta cheese

Makes 12 muffins, each:
Cal: 56, F: 2.5g, C: 2g (0.5g fiber) P: 6.5g

Enjoy in 45 minutes
Prep time: 15   Cook time: 25

Master Your Macros

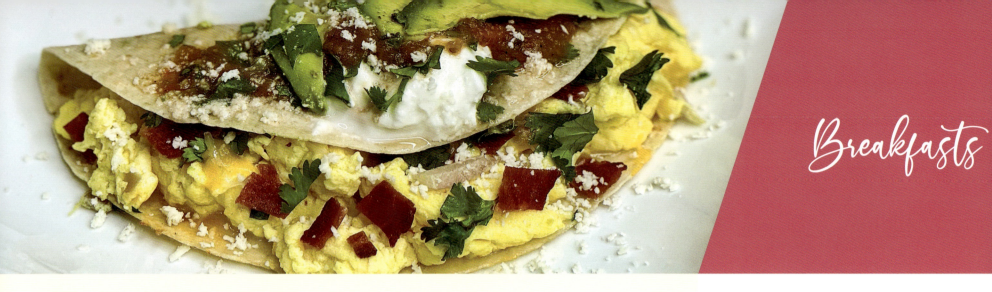

Loaded Breakfast Quesadilla

1. Spray a pan with non-stick spray and add onion. Cook over medium heat stirring occasionally until softened.
2. Whisk together egg, egg whites and 1 tbsp Greek yogurt in a medium bowl. Pour egg mixture into the pan over low-medium heat. Drag the eggs with a spatula to create curds. When the eggs are almost cooked to your liking, remove from the stove.
3. Spray pan with non-stick spray and assemble quesadilla: place 2 tbsp shredded Mexican cheese on bottom of 1/2 side of tortilla. Add scrambled eggs, chopped bacon, remaining shredded cheese, sprinkle cilantro and fold the tortilla in half.
4. Cook over medium heat until the bottom of the tortilla is golden, about 1-2 minutes. Spray the top of the tortilla with non-stick spray and flip to cook the other side.
5. Serve warm, topped with 1 tbsp Greek yogurt, sprinkle of cilantro, salsa and avocado.

Ingredients:
- 1 large egg (50g)
- 1/4 cup (60g) liquid egg whites
- 1 slice Godshalls Fully Cooked Uncured Turkey Bacon, diced
- 2 tbsp (6g) red onion, chopped
- 2 tbsp (30g) 0% plain Greek yogurt
- 1 Xtreme Wellness low carb tortilla
- 1/4 cup (28g) reduced-fat Mexican shredded cheese
- 2 tbsp (4g) cilantro, chopped
- 1/8 medium avocado (19g), sliced
- Salsa or Hot sauce for serving

Makes 1 quesadilla:
Cal: 318, F: 16g, C: 25g (14g fiber), P: 31g

Enjoy in 15 minutes
Prep time: 10   Cook time: 5

Master Your Macros

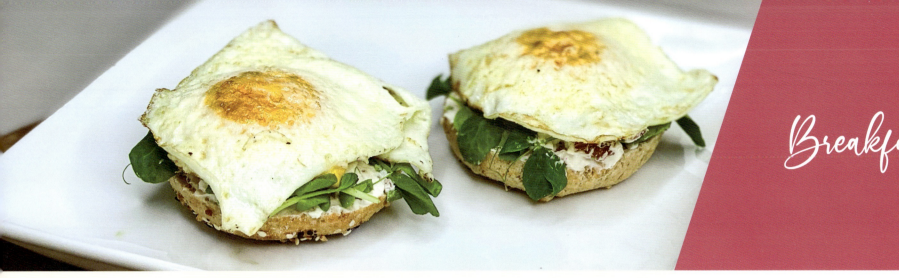

Egg & Bacon Cream Cheese Bagels

1. Prepare 'Everything Protein Bagels' per instructions on page 162.
2. Cook eggs to your liking. I chose fried eggs.
3. Mix bacon cream cheese ingredients in a bowl.
4. Assemble each half of bagel with 1/8 cream cheese mixture, greens and 1 egg. Enjoy!

Bagels:
+ See 'Everything Protein Bagels' recipe in the breads section

Bacon Cream Cheese:
+ 8oz. (224g) fat-free cream cheese, softened
+ 1/4 cup (26g) green onion, diced
+ 4 slices Godshalls Fully Cooked Uncured Turkey Bacon, diced
+ 1 tsp (1g) minced onion

Sandwich:
+ 4 'Everything Protein Bagels' cut in half
+ 8 large eggs (400g)
+ Arugula or greens of choice

Makes 8 servings:
Cal: 208, F: 6g, C: 21g (2g fiber), P: 17g

Enjoy in 10 minutes
Prep time: 5   Cook time: 5

Master Your Macros

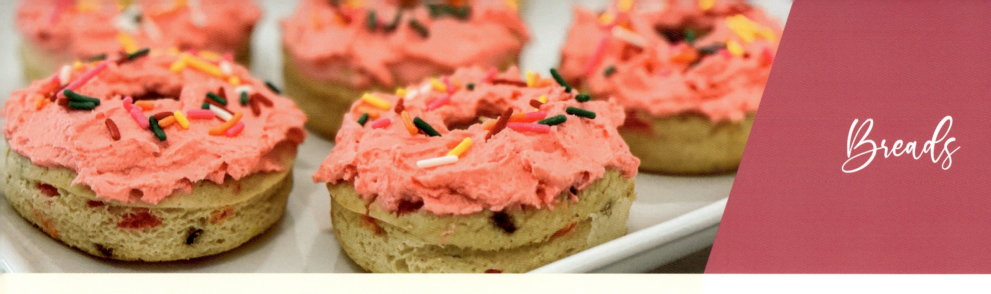

Rainbow Sprinkle Protein Donuts

1. Preheat oven to 350°F and coat 6 donut pan mold with non-stick spray.
2. Combine all ingredients in a medium sized bowl and mix until smooth.
3. Divide and pour batter in donut pan and bake for 15-20 minutes.
4. Mix frosting ingredients while donuts are baking.
5. Let donuts cool and top with frosting and sprinkles.

Ingredients:
- 1/2 cup (53g) Kodiak Cakes buttermilk flapjack & waffle mix
- 31g (1 scoop) Quest Vanilla Milkshake protein powder
- 2 tbsp (14g) coconut flour
- 1 tsp (4g) vanilla extract
- 1/4 cup (60g) liquid egg whites
- 3/4 cup (180mL) unsweetened cashew/almond milk
- 1/2 tsp (3g) baking powder
- 1 tbsp (12g) Swerve granular sugar substitute
- 6g rainbow sprinkles

Frosting:
- 1/2 cup (120g) 0% plain Greek yogurt
- 1 tbsp (12g) Swerve granular sugar substitute
- 1 tbsp (4g) vanilla sugar-free pudding mix
- Rainbow sprinkles and a drop or two of red food coloring to make it pink!

Makes 6 donuts, each:
Cal: 92, F: 1.5g, C: 10.5g (2g fiber), P: 9g

Enjoy in 35 minutes
Prep time: 15   Cook time: 20

Master Your Macros

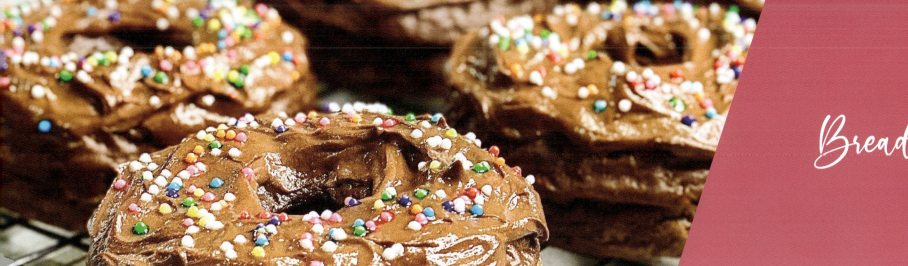

Breads

Double Chocolate Protein Donuts

1. Preheat oven to 350°F and coat a 6-mold donut pan with non-stick spray.
2. Mix wet and dry ingredients in separate bowls.
3. Combine wet and dry ingredients in a medium bowl and mix until smooth.
4. Divide and pour batter in donut pan and bake for 15-20 minutes.
5. Mix chocolate frosting ingredients while donuts are baking.
6. Let donuts cool, top with chocolate frosting and enjoy!

Ingredients:
- 60g (2 scoops) Quest Chocolate Milkshake protein powder
- 1/4 cup (26g) Kodiak Cakes buttermilk flapjack & waffle mix
- 1 large egg (50g)
- 1/4 cup (60g) liquid egg whites
- 1/4 cup (60g) canned pumpkin
- 1/4 cup (60g) unsweetened applesauce
- 1/4 cup (60mL) unsweetened cashew/almond milk
- 2 tbsp (10g) unsweetened cocoa powder
- 1 tsp (4g) baking powder

Chocolate Protein Icing:
- 15g (1/2 scoop) Quest Chocolate Milkshake Protein Powder
- 1/4 cup (60g) 0% plain Greek yogurt
- 2 tbsp (34g) Hershey's lite chocolate syrup

Makes 6 donuts, each:
Cal: 108, F: 1, C: 10.3 (2.5g fiber), P: 13.8g

Enjoy in 35 minutes
Prep time: **15**   Cook time: **20**

Master Your Macros

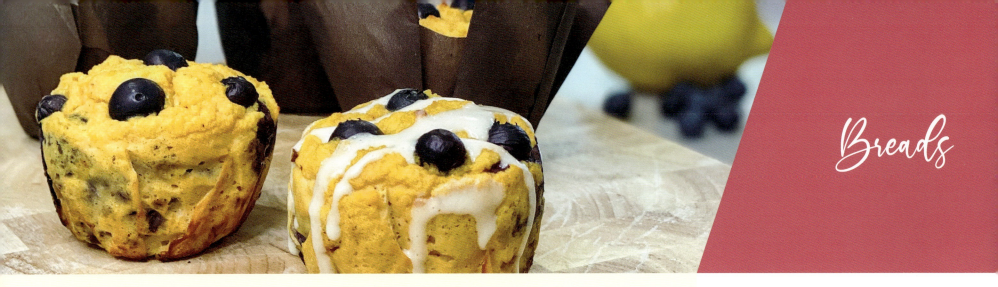

Blueberry Lemon Protein Muffins with Lemon Icing Drizzle

1. Preheat oven to 350°F and coat a 6-mold muffin pan mold with non-stick spray or parchment liners.
2. Mix wet and dry ingredients in separate bowls. Leave blueberries aside.
3. Combine wet and dry ingredients in a medium and mix until smooth. Fold in blueberries.
4. Divide and pour batter in muffin pan and bake for 24-28 minutes. Slightly undercooked is better than overcooked.
5. Let cool, drizzle icing and enjoy!

Makes 6 muffins, each:
Cal: 112 F: 1.5g, C: 10g (3g fiber), P: 13g

Enjoy in 45 minutes
Prep time: 20　Cook time: 25

Ingredients:
- 62g (2 scoops) Quest Vanilla Milkshake protein powder
- 1/4 cup (28g) coconut flour
- 1 large egg (50g)
- 1/4 cup (60g) liquid egg whites
- 1/4 cup (60mL) unsweetened cashew/almond milk
- 1/4 cup (60g) canned pumpkin
- 1/4 cup (60g) unsweetened applesauce
- 2 tbsp (7g) lemon sugar-free pudding mix
- 1 tsp (4g) vanilla extract
- 1 tsp (4g) baking powder
- 1/2 cup fresh blueberries (74g)

Lemon Protein Icing:
- 15g (1/2 scoop) Quest Vanilla Milkshake Protein Powder
- 1 tbsp (15mL) unsweetened cashew/almond milk
- 1 tsp (4g) Swerve confectioners powdered sugar substitute
- 1 tsp (4g) lemon juice

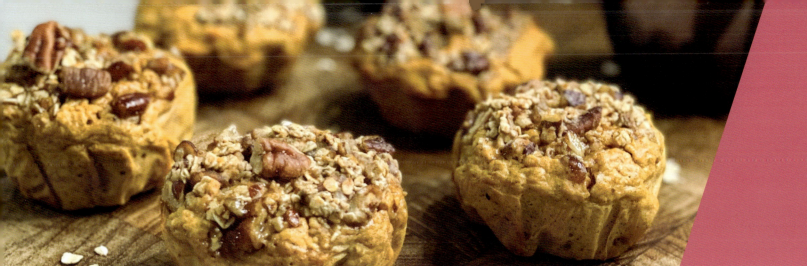

Pumpkin Oatmeal Muffins with Candied Pecan Streusel

1. Preheat oven to 350°F and spray a 12-muffin tin with non-stick spray.
2. Mash the banana with a fork and mix wet ingredients together.
3. Add dry ingredients to the bowl and mix thoroughly.
4. Use a large spoon to transfer the batter to the muffin tin or molds.
5. Mix the streusel ingredients in a small bowl and distribute evenly over the top of the muffins.
6. Bake for 15-20 minutes, or until a toothpick comes out clean. Enjoy!

Ingredients:
- 62g (2 scoops) Quest Vanilla Milkshake protein powder
- 3/4 cup (60g) oat flour
- 3/4 cup (180g) liquid egg whites
- 1/2 cup (120g) canned pumpkin
- 1/4 cup (60mL) sugar-free maple syrup
- 1 medium overripe banana (118g), mashed
- 2 tbsp (24g) Swerve granular sugar substitute
- 1 tsp (2g) pumpkin pie spice
- 1/2 tsp (2g) baking powder

Candied Pecan Streusel:
- 2 tbsp (30mL) sugar-free maple syrup
- 2 tbsp (24g) Swerve brown sugar substitute
- 2 tbsp (10g) quick oats
- 1/4 cup (30g) chopped pecans

Makes 12 muffins, each:
Cal: 83, F: 2.5g, C: 11g (3g fiber), P: 6.5g

Enjoy in 45 minutes
Prep time: 20 Cook time: 25

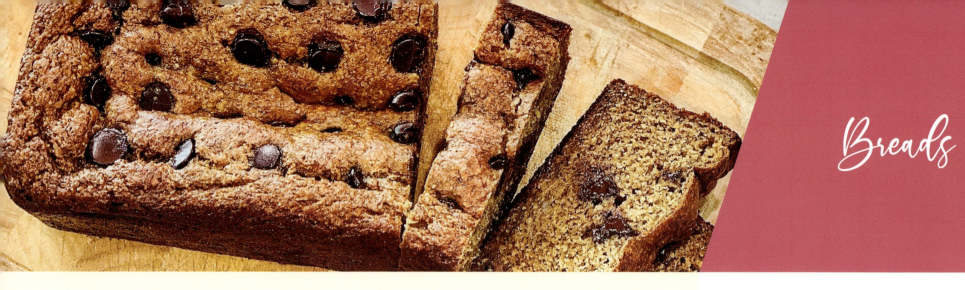

Banana Chocolate Chip Protein Bread

1. Preheat oven to 350°F and spray a bread pan with non-stick spray.
2. Mix wet and dry ingredients in separate bowls, except chocolate chips.
3. Mix wet and dry ingredients together and pour in the bread pan. Top with chocolate chips.
4. Bake for 40-45 minutes. Slightly undercooked is better than overcooked.
5. Let cool for about 10-15 minutes, slice into 8 pieces, and enjoy!

Ingredients:
- 1 cup (80g) oat flour
- 62g (2 scoops) Quest Cinnamon Cereal protein powder
- 3 overripe medium bananas (354g), mashed
- 1/2 cup (96g) Swerve granular sugar substitute
- 1/4 cup (60g) 0% plain Greek yogurt
- 1/4 cup (60g) unsweetened applesauce
- 1 large egg (50g)
- 1 tsp (4g) baking soda
- 1 tsp (4g) baking powder
- 1 tsp (4g) cinnamon
- 1 tsp (4g) vanilla extract
- 2 tbsp (20g) Lily's semi-sweet chocolate chips

Makes 8 slices, each:
Cal: 119, F: 2g, C: 17.5g (2g fiber), P: 7.5g

Enjoy in 70 minutes
Prep time: **25**   Cook time: **45**

Master Your Macros

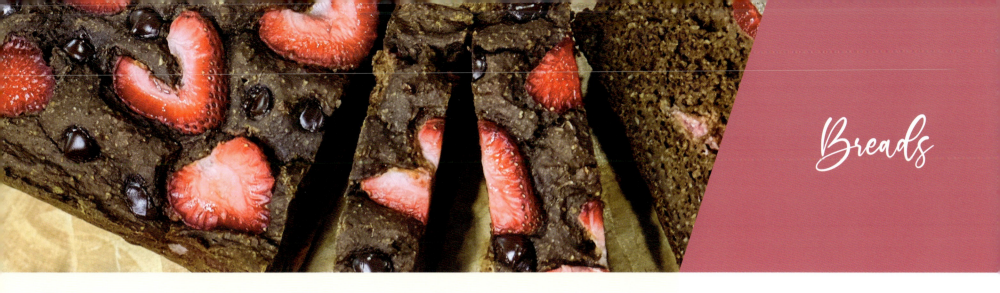

Chocolate Strawberry Protein Bread

1. Preheat oven to 350°F and spray a bread pan with non-stick spray.
2. Mix dry and wet ingredients in separate bowls, leaving out strawberries and chocolate chips.
3. Combine wet and dry ingredients and fold in 2/3 strawberries and 1/2 of the chocolate chips.
4. Spread mix in bread pan and top with remaining chocolate chips and strawberries.
5. Bake for 40-45 minutes. Slightly undercooked is better than overcooked.
6. Let cool for about 10-15 minutes, slice into 8 pieces and enjoy!

Ingredients:
- 1 cup (80g) oat flour
- 60g (2 scoops) Quest Chocolate Milkshake protein powder
- 1/2 cup (96g) Swerve granular sugar substitute
- 1 tbsp (5g) unsweetened cocoa powder
- 1 tbsp (10g) whole flax seed
- 1 tsp (4g) baking soda
- 1 tsp (4g) baking powder
- 1 cup (240g) canned pumpkin
- 1/4 cup (60g) 0% plain Greek yogurt
- 1/4 cup (60g) unsweetened applesauce
- 1/4 cup (60g) water
- 1/4 cup (40g) Lily's semi-sweet chocolate chips
- 1/2 cup strawberries (100g), diced

Makes 8 slices, each:
Cal: 114, F: 3g, C: 16.5g (5g fiber), P: 9g

Enjoy in 70 minutes
Prep time: 25   Cook time: 45

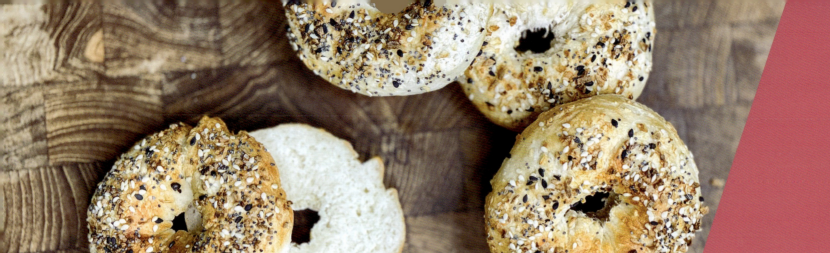

Breads

Everything Protein Bagels

1. Combine Kodiak cakes, baking powder, Greek yogurt, salt and 2 tbsp egg whites to a bowl and mix until you have a dough ball. Use your hands to knead the dough until all the flour is absorbed.
2. Separate into 4 equal sized pieces (about 90g each) then roll them out with your hands into a tube. Massage the ends together to form a bagel. If the dough is too sticky, sprinkle a little Kodiak Cakes flour on the surface.
3. Drizzle 1/2 tbsp egg white on top of each formed bagel and sprinkle Everything But The Bagel seasoning on top.
4. Cook in your air fryer basket at 350°F for 5-8 minutes, depending on how well done you want them.
5. Let them sit for 5-10 minutes to cool. Slice, top with cream cheese or other toppings of choice. Check out the Egg & Bacon Cream Cheese Bagels breakfast recipe! Enjoy.

Ingredients:
+ 1 1/2 cup + 3 tsp (180g) Kodiak Cakes Whole Wheat & Honey flapjack and waffle mix
+ 2 tsp (8g) baking powder
+ 2/3 cup (160g) plain 0% Greek yogurt
+ 4 tbsp (60g) liquid egg whites
+ 1/2 tsp (2g) salt
+ Everything But the Bagel seasoning

Makes 4 bagels, each:
Cal: 176, F: 1g, C: 33g (4g fiber), P: 11

Enjoy in 20 minutes
Prep time: **12**   Cook time: **8**

Master Your Macros

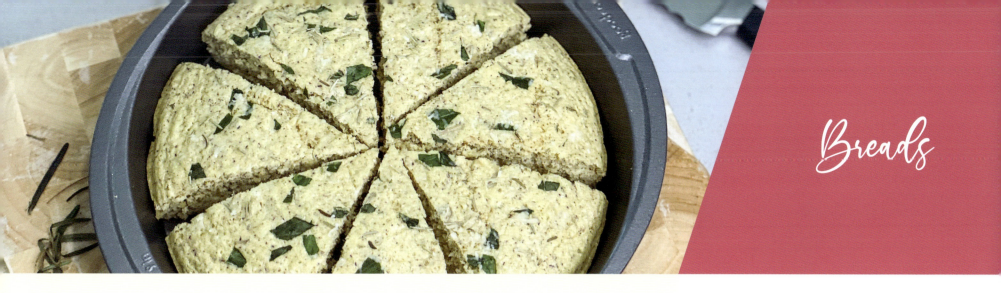

Rosemary Focaccia Protein Bread

1. Preheat oven to 325°F and spray 9-10" baking pan with non-stick spray.
2. Mix wet and dry ingredients separately, except parmesan cheese.
3. Combine wet and dry ingredients and pour batter into pan. Sprinkle parmesan cheese and a little extra rosemary on top.
4. Bake for 15 minutes, or until firm and a toothpick comes out clean. Best not to overcook!
5. Let cool, slice and enjoy!

Ingredients:
+ 1 1/2 cups (360g) liquid egg whites
+ 1 tsp (5mL) extra-virgin olive oil
+ 1 cup (80g) oat flour
+ 1/4 cup (20g) whole psyllium husks
+ 3/4 cup (2 1/3 scoop) ISO100 unflavored whey protein powder
+ 2 tsp (10g) baking powder
+ 1/2 tsp (3g) sea salt
+ 1 tsp (5g) minced garlic
+ 1 tbsp (1g) dried rosemary
+ 1 tsp (>1g) dried oregano
+ 2 tsp (>1g) fresh basil, chopped
+ 1 tbsp (14g) parmesan

Makes 10 slices, each:
Cal: 87, F: 1g, C: 7.5g (3g fiber), P: 11

Enjoy in 35 minutes
Prep time: **20**   Cook time: **15**

Master Your Macros

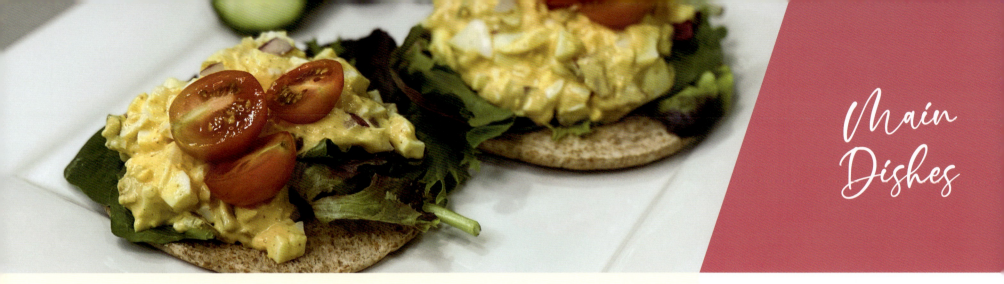

Main Dishes

Egg Salad Slimwich

1. Cut open hard-boiled eggs. Place four egg yolks in a bowl. Dice egg whites into small chunks and set aside.
2. Add yogurt, mustard and relish to bowl and mash with egg yolks until completely mixed.
3. Fold in diced egg whites and red onion.
4. Spread half of the egg mixture on top of one sandwich thin and top with mixed greens and tomatoes.

Ingredients:
+ 4 large hard-boiled eggs (200g)
+ 2 large hard-boiled egg whites (60g)
+ 2 tbsp (30g) 0% plain Greek yogurt
+ 1 tbsp (15g) pickle relish
+ 1 tbsp (15g) spicy mustard
+ 2 tbsp (6g) red onion, chopped
+ Diced cherry tomatoes and mixed greens for serving
+ 2 whole wheat sandwich thins

Makes 2 sandwiches, each:
Cal: 307, F:11g, C: 28g (5.5g fiber), P: 32g

Enjoy in 10 minutes

Master Your Macros

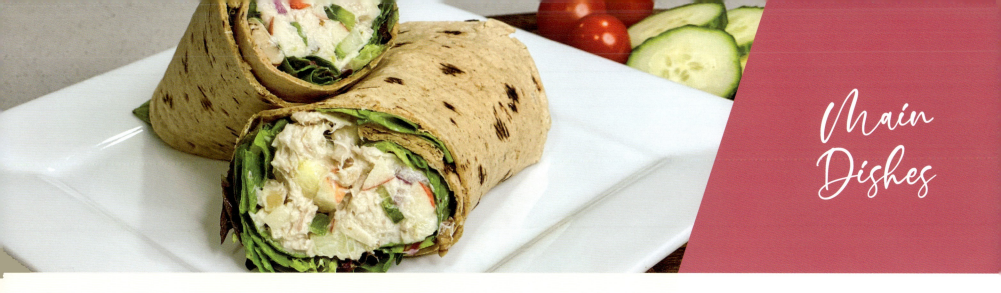

Apple Walnut Tuna Salad Wrap

1. In a bowl mix tuna, yogurt, apple, celery, walnuts, onion and relish.
2. Top Flatout flatbread with 1/2 mixed greens and 1/2 tuna mixture, wrap and enjoy!

Ingredients:
+ 5oz. (113g) albacore tuna in water, drained
+ 1/3 cup (80g) 0% plain Greek yogurt
+ 1/2 cup (60g) red apple, diced
+ 1/4 cup (25g) celery, chopped
+ 1/4 cup (30g) walnuts, chopped
+ 2 tbsp (15g) onion, chopped
+ 2 tbsp (15g) sweet pickle relish
+ 1/2 cup (38g) mixed greens
+ 2 Flatout light flatbreads

Makes 2 wraps, each:
Cal: 329, F:12g, C:30g (11g fiber), P:29.5

Enjoy in 10 minutes

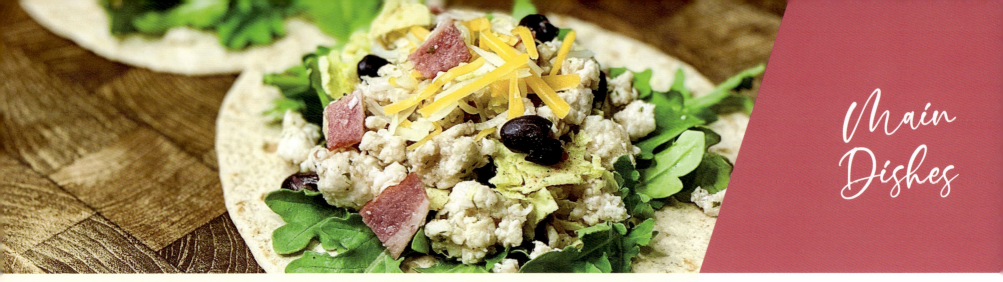

Chicken, Bacon & Ranch Street Tacos

1. Cook the bacon in a large skillet over medium-high heat. Transfer the cooked bacon to a paper towel, drain the remaining grease, and dice into small pieces.
2. Add the ground chicken to the pan and cook until no pink remains.
3. Add the ranch seasoning, bacon, black beans and Greek yogurt to the cooked ground chicken. Stir well and let simmer for 5 minutes to allow flavors to merge.
4. Place some arugula on the bottom of each tortilla. Top with 1/8 of the meat mixture and cheese.
5. Open bag of Quest chips and crush chips inside the bag. Top each taco with 1/8 bag of chips. This adds a nice crunch and boost of ranch flavor to the tacos! Enjoy!

Ingredients:
- 16oz. 97% lean ground chicken breast
- 4 slices Smoked Turkey Bacon, diced
- 3 tbsp (16g) ranch seasoning mix
- 1/2 cup (130g) reduced-sodium black beans, drained and rinsed.
- 1/2 cup (120g) 0% plain Greek yogurt
- 1/4 cup (28g) reduced-fat Mexican blend cheese, shredded
- 8 Mission Carb Balance Street Tacos tortillas
- 1 bag (32g) Quest ranch tortilla style protein chips
- 1/2 cup (38g) arugula

Main Dishes

Makes 8 street tacos, each:
Cal: 170, F:5.5g, C:14g (9.5g fiber), P:22.5g

Enjoy in 30 minutes
Prep time: **10** Cook time: **20**

Master Your Macros

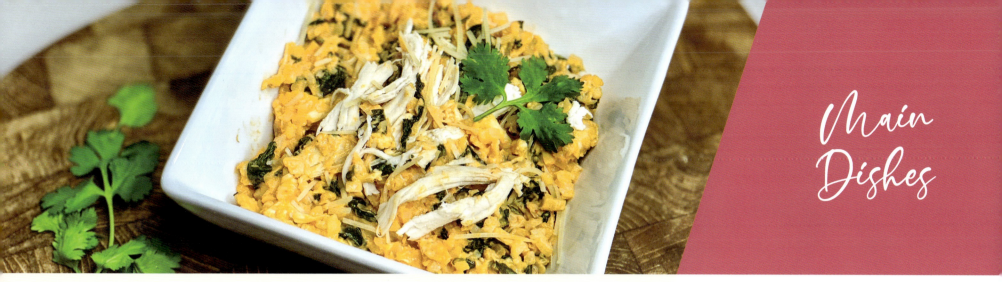

Chicken & Cauliflower Cheesy Rice

1. Steam cauliflower rice in the microwave. When done, open the bag and squeeze excess juice from rice.
2. Spray a large pan with non-stick spray, add spinach and garlic to cook.
3. In a bowl mix the cheddar cheese powder, Greek yogurt and almond milk to make a creamy cheese spread.
4. Add the cooked rice, chicken, cheese and sriracha to the pan. Mix thoroughly.
5. Reduce the heat to low, stir and let simmer for 5 minutes to fully incorporate.
6. Serve 1/4 mixture topped with 1 tbsp parmesan cheese and enjoy!

Ingredients:
- 16oz. cooked and diced rotisserie chicken breast
- 1 bag (149g) raw baby spinach
- 1 bag (283g) frozen microwavable cauliflower rice
- 1 1/2 tbsp (8g) minced garlic
- 2 tbsp (30g) sriracha chili hot sauce (more or less depending on spice preference).
- 1/2 cup (56g) Anthony's Cheddar Powder
- 1/2 cup (120g) 0% plain Greek yogurt
- 2 tbsp (30g) unsweetened cashew/almond milk
- 4 tbsp (28g) parmesan cheese

Makes 4 servings, each:
Cal: 240, F: 7.5g, C: 11g (2.5g fiber), P: 28.5g

Enjoy in 25 minutes
Prep time: 10   Cook time: 15

Master Your Macros

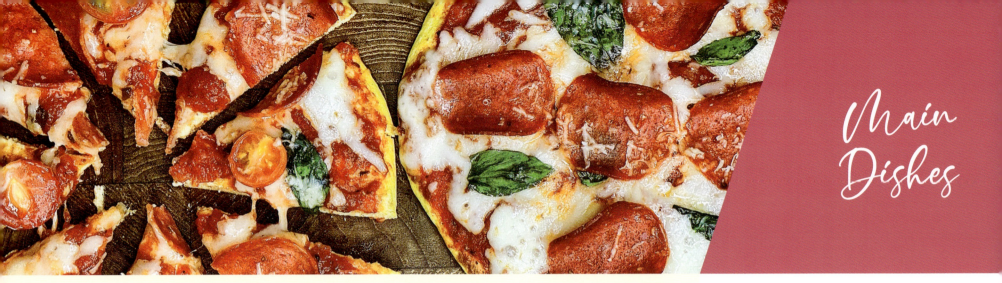

Main Dishes

Pepperoni Protein Pizza

1. Add crust ingredients into a bowl and whisk together until smooth.
2. Preheat oven to 400°F and stovetop pan on 6/10 heat. Spray the pan with nonstick cooking spray and add half the crust batter to the middle of the pan.
3. Spread the batter around in the pan to flatten the batter and form the circular shape of your crust. Add a cover to the pan and cook for 2-3 minutes.
4. Spray the top of the crust with nonstick cooking spray and flip it over. Press edges down with the spatula to prevent curling. Cook on that side for another 2-3 minutes. Repeat this process with the second half of your batter.
5. Place crusts on a pizza pan and split the toppings on each crust.
6. Place in the oven for about 8 minutes. Enjoy!

Crust Ingredients:
+ 1 cup (240g) liquid egg whites
+ 1/4 cup (24g) coconut flour
+ 1/2 tsp (1g) garlic powder
+ 1/2 tsp (1g) McCormick Tasty Cheesy seasoning mix
+ Pinch of Sea Salt

Toppings:
+ 1/2 cup (113g) Classico Tomato & Basil sauce
+ 6 tbsp (85g) shredded mozzarella
+ 1 tbsp (15g) shredded parmesan
+ 1oz. (16g) reduced-fat turkey pepperoni
+ Fresh basil leaves

Makes 2 pizzas, each:
Cal: 264, F:10g, C:12g (5g fiber), P: 25.5g

Enjoy in 35 minutes
Prep time: **15**   Cook time: **20**

Master Your Macros

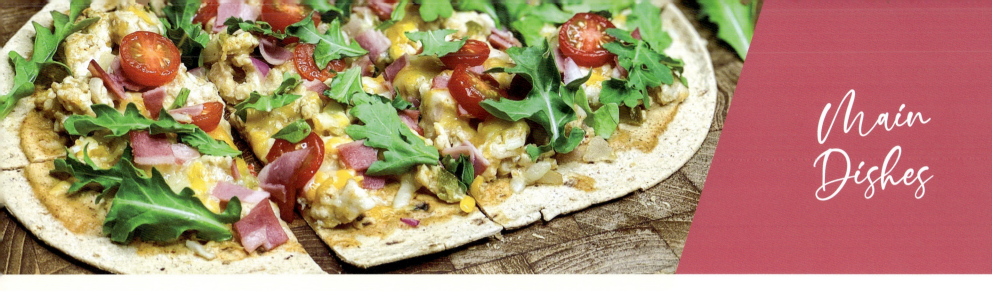

Turkey Bacon Cheeseburger Flatbread

1. Preheat oven to 350°F.
2. Combine ketchup, Greek yogurt, and mustard.
3. Spray skillet with non-stick spray and cook onion until translucent. Add ground turkey and cook until no pink remains.
4. Stir in jalapeño, 1/2 cup shredded cheese and half of the ketchup mixture. Cook over medium heat until heated through.
5. Brush each flatbread with 1/4 of reserved ketchup mixture and top with 1/4 cooked ground turkey mixture, cheese and 1 slice of diced turkey bacon and diced tomatoes.
6. Bake for 5-6 minutes or until the cheese is melted and flatbread is slightly crisp. Remove from oven, top with arugula, slice and enjoy!

Ingredients:
- 16oz. 99% lean ground turkey
- 4 slices Oscar Mayer cooked smoked turkey bacon, chopped
- 1/3 cup (75g) no sugar added ketchup
- 1/3 cup (80g) 0% plain Greek yogurt
- 3 tbsp (45g) spicy brown mustard
- 1/4 cup (60g) jalapeño, chopped
- 1 cup (56g) reduced-fat shredded cheese
- 1/2 cup (60g) red onion, diced
- Cherry tomatoes, diced
- Arugula
- 4 Flatout light original flatbreads

Makes 4 flatbreads, each:
Cal: 370, F: 10.5g, C: 29g (11g fiber), P: 44.5g

Enjoy in 20 minutes
Prep time: **15** Cook time: **5**

Master Your Macros

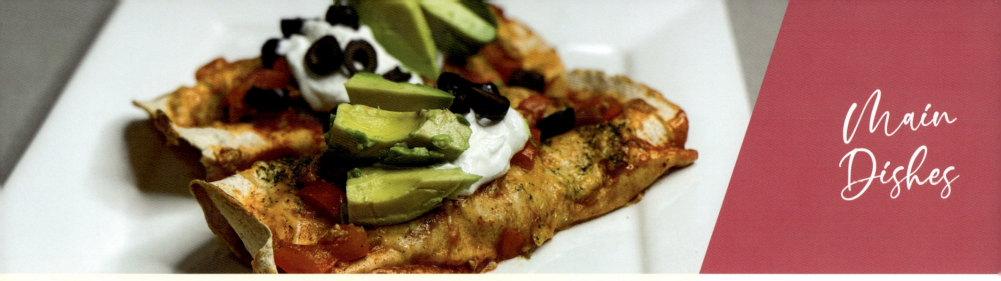

Turkey Enchiladas

1. Preheat oven to 375°F.
2. Spray baking dish with non-stick spray, spread 1/4 enchilada sauce along bottom.
3. Cook bell pepper in a skillet until it's soft. Add ground turkey, green chilies, chili powder and 1/2 the enchilada sauce. Simmer until the meat is browned.
4. Divide mixture between 6 tortillas. Wrap and set inside the baking dish.
5. Top enchiladas with remaining enchilada sauce, cheese and parsley and bake for 20-25 minutes.
6. Garnish enchiladas with Greek yogurt, diced avocado and olives.

Crust Ingredients:
+ 16oz. 99% lean ground turkey
+ 2 medium bell pepper (240g), diced
+ 19oz. (538g) enchilada sauce
+ 1 1/2 tsp (1g) chili powder
+ 4oz. (113g) diced green chiles
+ 1oz. (30g) sliced black olives
+ 1/2 cup (112g) shredded Mexican blend cheese
+ 1 tsp (1g) parsley
+ 3/4 cup (180g) 0% plain Greek yogurt
+ 1 1/2 small avocado (225g), sliced
+ 6 low carb tortillas

Makes 6 servings, each:
Cal: 319, F: 13g, C: 31g (15g fiber), P: 28g

Enjoy in 40 minutes
Prep time: **20**   Cook time: **20**

Master Your Macros

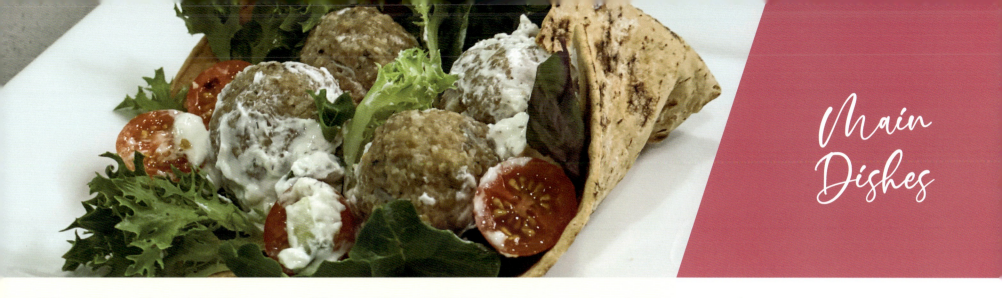

Main Dishes

Greek Meatball Wrap w/ Tzatziki Yogurt Sauce

1. Preheat oven to 350°F and line a baking sheet with parchment paper.
2. In a large bowl, combine ground turkey, egg whites, breadcrumbs, onion, garlic, parsley, oregano, salt, pepper and mix well with your hands.
3. Form into 16 golf sized meatballs, place evenly across baking sheet and bake for 30 minutes.
4. In a bowl mix Tzatziki Herb Yogurt Sauce ingredients.
5. Spread 1/4 yogurt sauce on one Flatout flatbread, top with lettuce, tomato, onion and 4 meatballs. Wrap tightly and enjoy!

Ingredients:
+ 16oz. 93% lean ground turkey
+ 2 tbsp (30g) liquid egg whites
+ 2 tbsp (14g) parmesan cheese
+ 1/4 cup (28g) Italian breadcrumbs
+ 1/4 cup (14g) onion, chopped
+ 1 tsp (5g) minced garlic
+ 1 tsp (1g) dried parsley
+ Pinch of dried oregano and black pepper
+ 4 Flatout light flatbreads
+ Sliced grape tomatoes, diced onion and mixed greens for serving

Tzatziki Yogurt Sauce:
+ 1 cup (240g) 0% plain Greek yogurt
+ 1/2 cup (28g) chopped cucumber
+ 1/2 tbsp (14g) lemon juice
+ 1 tsp (1g) dried dill weed
+ 1 tsp (5g) white vinegar
+ 1 tsp (5g) minced garlic

Makes 4 wraps, each:
Cal: 360, F:11g, C: 33g (11.5g fiber), P: 38.5

Enjoy in 50 minutes
Prep time: **20**   Cook time: **30**

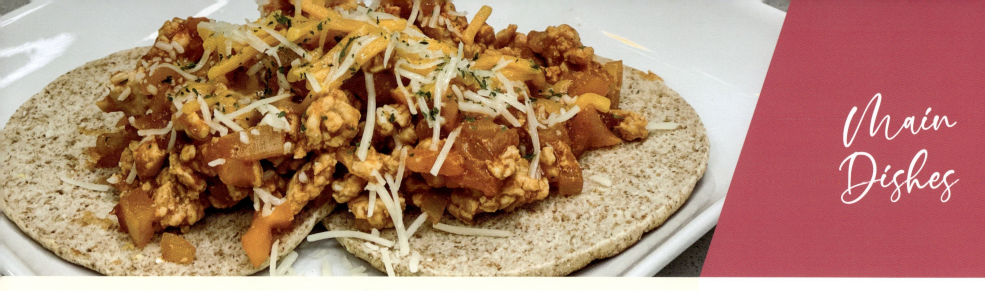

Main Dishes

Turkey Sloppy (Thin) Joes

1. In a small bowl mix together ketchup, Worcestershire sauce, sugar-free maple syrup, spicy brown mustard, minced garlic and black pepper.
2. Cook bell pepper and onion in a skillet over medium heat until soft.
3. Add ground turkey to skillet and cook until it begins to brown.
4. Stir in sauce and spice mixture, reduce heat and simmer for 10 minutes.
5. Remove the lid for about 5 minutes, or until the mixture thickens.
6. Serve 1/4 mixture with 1/4 mozzarella cheese on top of one sandwich thin.

Ingredients:
+ 16oz. 99% lean ground turkey
+ 1 medium bell pepper (120g), diced
+ 1 cup (60g) onion, chopped
+ 3/4 cup (180g) no-sugar added ketchup
+ 1 tbsp (15mL) Worcestershire sauce
+ 1 tbsp (15mg) spicy brown mustard
+ 1 tbsp (15g) minced garlic
+ 1/4 cup (60mL) sugar-free maple syrup
+ 1/4 tsp (1g) ground black pepper
+ 1/4 cup (28g) shredded mozzarella cheese
+ 4 whole wheat sandwich slims

Makes 4 servings, each:
Cal: 283, F:3.5g, C:33g (7g fiber), P:33g

Enjoy in 30 minutes
Prep time: 10   Cook time: 20

Master Your Macros

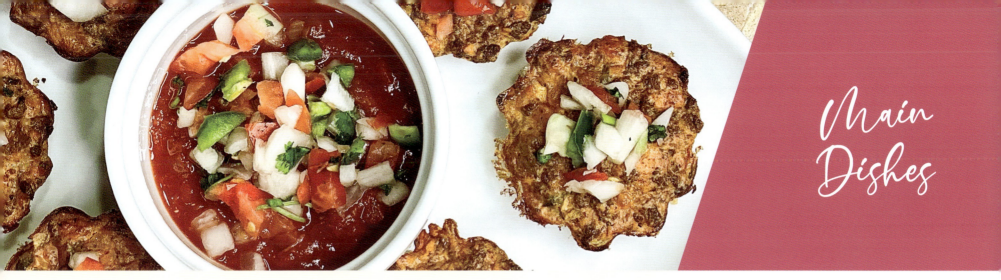

Main Dishes

Taco Fiesta Bites

1. Preheat oven to 400°F and spray a 12-muffin pan with non-stick spray.
2. Cook the ground beef over medium heat. Use a spatula to finely crumble the beef. Drain excess fat.
3. Add taco seasoning to beef and remove from heat.
4. Open Quest Nacho Chip bags and crush the bag with your hands to break the chips into small crumbs. Fold crumbs into beef mixture.
5. Mix remaining ingredients in a separate bowl and add into the cooked beef.
6. Spoon the mixture into 12 muffin mold.
7. Bake for 22-25 minutes or until the taco bites are cooked in the center.

Ingredients:
+ 16oz. 96% lean ground beef
+ 1 packet (30g) reduced-sodium taco seasoning
+ 64g (2 bags) Quest nacho cheese protein chips, crushed
+ 1 cup (240g) liquid egg whites
+ 1/2 cup (120g) 0% plain Greek yogurt
+ 1 cup (112g) shredded cheddar cheese
+ 1/4 cup (60g) salsa
+ 2oz. (57g) sliced jalapeños. Provides a nice heat. Reduce or omit based on spicy preference.

Makes 12 servings, each:
Cal: 115, F: 4g, C: 5.5g (1g fiber), P: 15.5

Enjoy in 40 minutes
Prep time: 15   Cook time: 25

Master Your Macros

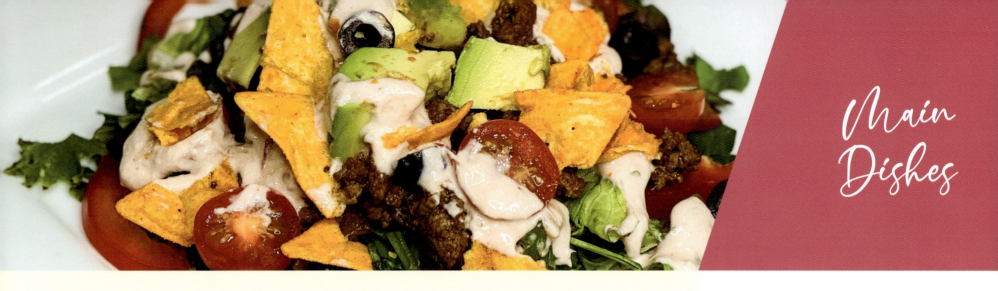

Beef Nacho Salad

1. Cook beef over medium heat until brown, drain excess fat.
2. Add taco seasoning, onion, jalapenos and water. Reduce heat and let simmer for 5 minutes.
3. Serve 1/4 meat mixture on top 2 cups mixed greens.
4. Top each salad with 1/4 bell peppers, tomatoes, olives, avocado and Quest tortilla chips, dressing and enjoy!

Ingredients:
+ 16oz. 96% lean ground beef
+ 1 packet (30g) reduced-sodium taco seasoning
+ 3/4 cup (180g) water
+ 1/2 cup (30g) red onion, chopped
+ 1 tbsp (30g) diced jalapeño (more or less depending on how spicy you like)
+ 1/2 medium red bell pepper (60g), sliced
+ 16 grape tomatoes, sliced (100g)
+ 1 small avocado, sliced (150g)
+ 2 tbsp (22g) sliced black olives
+ 8 cups chopped mixed greens (600g)
+ 32g (1 bag) Quest nacho cheese protein chips

Dressing:
+ 1/2 cup (120mL) salsa
+ 3/4 cup (180g) 0% plain Greek yogurt

Makes 4 salads, each:
Cal: 337, F:12g, C:16g (3g fiber), P:35.5

Enjoy in 25 minutes
Prep time: **15**   Cook time: **10**

Master Your Macros

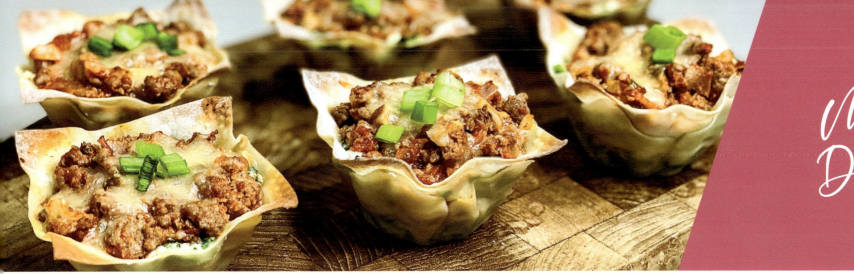

Main Dishes

Cheesy Beef & Spinach Lasagna Cups

1. Preheat oven to 375°F and spray a 12-cup muffin pan with non-stick spray.
2. In a large skillet, cook beef over medium-high heat until browned then drain excess fat. Add onion and mushrooms. Cook until onions become slightly translucent.
3. Add marinara sauce and 1 1/2 tsp. garlic.
4. In a bowl mix spinach, basil, ricotta cheese, egg whites and 1/2 tsp. garlic.
5. Press a wonton wrapper into the bottom and sides of each muffin mold and evenly distribute half of the spinach-ricotta mixture (~1 tbsp. each), top with half of the beef mixture (~1 1/2 tbsp. each). Smooth out and lightly press down the tops. Top with half of the mozzarella cheese.
6. Place another wonton wrapper into each cup, lightly pressing it down and along the sides, letting the edges fall over the pan. Repeat ingredients in step 5.
7. Bake until spinach-ricotta mixture is hot, mozzarella has melted, and wrapper edges have browned, about 10-15 minutes.

Ingredients:
+ 16oz. 96% lean ground beef
+ 1 tsp. (2g) black pepper
+ 1 cup (150g) onion, chopped
+ 1/2 cup (40g) mushrooms, chopped
+ 1 1/2 cups (335g) marinara sauce
+ 2 tsp (10g) minced garlic
+ 2 tsp (<1g) fresh basil, chopped
+ 8oz. (227g) frozen chopped spinach, thawed, excess water drained
+ 1 1/4 cups (310g) low-fat ricotta cheese
+ 1/4 cup (60g) liquid egg whites
+ 1 1/4 cups (140g) shredded part-skim mozzarella cheese
+ 24 small square wonton wrappers (in the refrigerated section next to the tofu)

Makes 12 cups, each:
Cal: 165, F: 5g, C: 14g (1.5g fiber), P: 16.5g

Enjoy in 50 minutes
Prep time: **35** Cook time: **15**

Master Your Macros

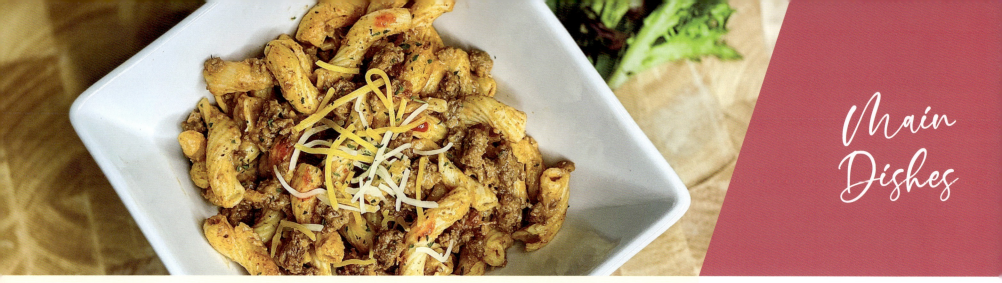

Main Dishes

Spicy Beef Mac & Cheese

1. Bring a pot of water to a boil to cook the pasta. Cooking one to two minutes short of package directions will help keep pasta from falling apart in step 7.
2. In a bowl mix the cheddar cheese powder, Greek yogurt and almond milk to make a creamy cheese spread.
3. Spray a large skillet with non-stick spray and cook beef over medium-high heat, chopping into small pieces with your spatula and drain excess fat once the beef is cooked.
4. Mix the spices in a small bowl and add to the top of the ground beef.
5. Add sriracha and mix thoroughly.
6. Reduce the heat to low and add the cheese mixture.
7. Add cooked pasta and reduce the heat to low, stir and let simmer for 5 minutes to fully incorporate. Enjoy!

Ingredients:
- 16oz. 96% lean ground beef
- 1 tsp (1g) chili powder
- 1 tsp (5g) minced garlic
- 1 tsp (1g) minced onion powder
- 1 tsp (1g) black pepper
- 2 tbsp (30g) sriracha chili hot sauce (more or less depending on spice preference)
- 1/2 cup (56g) Anthony's Cheddar Powder
- 1/2 cup (120g) 0% plain Greek yogurt
- 2 tbsp (30g) unsweetened cashew/almond milk
- 8oz. (227g) Banza Pasta Elbows

Makes 5 servings, each:
Cal: 340, F: 9.5g, C: 30g (4g fiber), P: 34.5g

Enjoy in 30 minutes
Prep time: **10**   Cook time: **20**

Master Your Macros

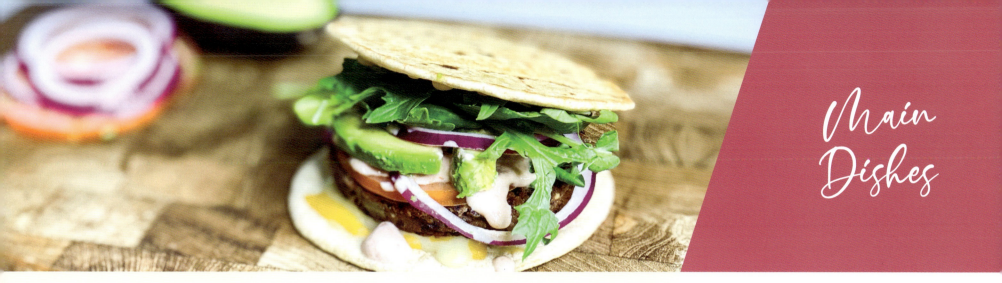

Black Bean Quesadilla Burgers

1. In a large bowl, use a potato masher or fork, to mash black beans until about half are still intact. Add remaining patty ingredients and mash to combine.
2. Form mixture into 3 balls and flatten into patties.
3. Spray a pan or griddle with non-stick spray and cook patties on medium heat for about 5 minutes each side, remove from heat.
4. Spray the pan or griddle with non-stick spray and place 2 tortillas with 1/4 cup cheese spread over the top. Let the tortilla crisp and the cheese melt before removing from heat.
5. Place one black bean burger patty on top one tortilla. Top with 1/3 of the sliced avocado, onion, greens, tomato and creamy salsa drizzle. Place the other tortilla on top. Enjoy!

Patty Ingredients:
- 15oz. (130g) black beans, rinsed and dried
- 1 bag (32g) Quest Nacho Cheese protein chips, crumbled
- 2oz. (56g) diced green chiles
- 1 tbsp (15g) sriracha
- 1 tbsp (15g) cilantro paste or chopped cilantro
- 2 tsp (10g) minced garlic
- 1 tsp (1g) cumin
- 1 tsp (1g) chili powder

Burger Ingredients:
- 6 Carb Balance Street Tacos tortillas
- 3/4 cup (84g) reduced-fat shredded 4-cheese mexican blend
- 1/2 medium avocado (30g), diced tomatoes, red onion and greens

Creamy Salsa Drizzle: Combine 1/2 cup (120g) 0% plain greek yogurt and 1/4 cup (60mL) salsa.

Makes 3 quesadilla burgers, each:
Cal: 416, F: 15g, C: 55g (29g fiber), P: 31g

Enjoy in 40 minutes
Prep time: 25 Cook time: 15

Master Your Macros

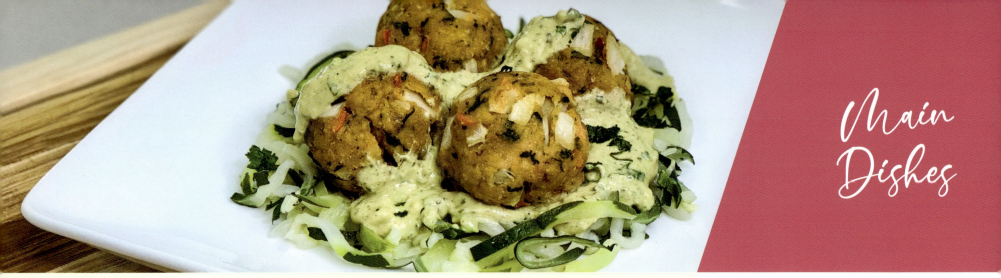

Avocado Cilantro Salmon Meatballs & Zucchini Spaghetti

1. Preheat oven to 350°F. Spray a large baking sheet with non-stick spray.
2. Place salmon in your food processor and pulse until finely ground, or see your market butcher for ground wild salmon.
3. Mix onion, breadcrumbs, cilantro, egg white, garlic, salt, pepper, paprika and oregano, then add your ground salmon. Thoroughly mix to combine.
4. Form salmon mixture into 12 golf-sized balls and place on your baking sheet.
5. Bake for 15-18 minutes, or until the meatballs are firm to the touch and cooked through.
6. Avocado Sauce: In a bowl, mash and combine the avocado, yogurt, garlic, lime juice, water, cilantro, chipotle powder, Chile powder, salt and pepper.
7. Dish 1 cup zucchini spirals, 4 meatballs and 1/3 Avocado Cilantro Sauce, enjoy!

Makes 3 servings, each:
Cal: 385, F: 16.7g, C: 15.5g (4.7g fiber), P:39g

Enjoy in 40 minutes
Prep time: **22**   Cook time: **18**

Meatball Ingredients:
- 1 lb (16oz.) skinless wild salmon, ground
- 1/2 cup (60g) onion, diced
- 1/4 cup (28g) plain panko breadcrumbs
- 3 tbsp (5g) cilantro, finely chopped
- 2 tbsp (30g) liquid egg whites
- 2 tsp (10g) minced garlic
- 1/2 tsp (2g) salt
- 1/2 tsp (2g) black pepper
- 1/2 tsp (2g) paprika
- 1/2 tsp (1/2g) dried oregano

Avocado Cilantro Sauce Ingredients:
- 1/2 medium avocado (60g)
- 1/4 cup (60g) 0% plain Greek yogurt
- 1 tsp (5g) minced garlic
- 1 tbsp (15g) lime juice
- 2 tbsp water
- 2 tbsp (3g) cilantro, finely chopped
- 1/4 tsp (<1g) ground chipotle
- 1/4 tsp (<1g) chili powder
- Salt and black pepper to taste
- 3 cups (510g) zucchini spirals prepared per package directions.

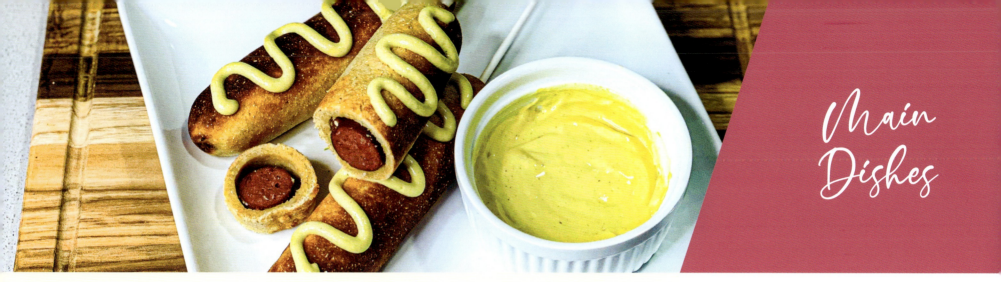

Protein Corn Dogs with Maple Dijon Mustard

1. Add Kodiak cakes mix, baking powder, Greek yogurt, and salt to a bowl and mix until you have a dough ball. Use your hands to knead the dough until all the flour is absorbed.
2. Separate into 4 equal sized pieces (about 90g each), then roll them into balls.
3. Between two pieces of parchment paper, roll each ball flat into a rectangle.
4. Wrap flattened dough around one hot dog and massage all edges together until the dog is sealed inside. Repeat with remaining three dough balls.
5. Cook corn dogs in your air fryer basket at 350°F for 8-10 minutes. Flip dog half way through.
6. While dogs cook, mix the Maple Dijon Mustard ingredients.
7. Let dogs sit for 5 minutes to cool. Insert stick (optional), and serve each dog with 1/4 mustard dip. Enjoy.

Ingredients:
+ 4 Durham Ranch 12oz. Uncured Bison with Beef Hot Dogs (or dogs of choice)
+ 1 1/2 cup + 3 tsp (180g) Kodiak Cakes Cornbread mix
+ 2 tsp (8g) baking powder
+ 2/3 cup (160g) 0% plain Greek yogurt
+ 1/2 tsp (2g) salt

Maple Dijon Mustard Dip:
+ 2 tbsp (30mL) sugar-free maple syrup
+ 2 tbsp (30g) yellow mustard
+ 1 tbsp (15g) dijon mustard
+ 1/4 cup (60g) 0% plain Greek yogurt

Makes 4 corn dogs, each:
Cal: 320, F: 7g, C: 36.5g (3g fiber), P: 28.5g

Enjoy in 20 minutes
Prep time: **10**   Cook time: **10**

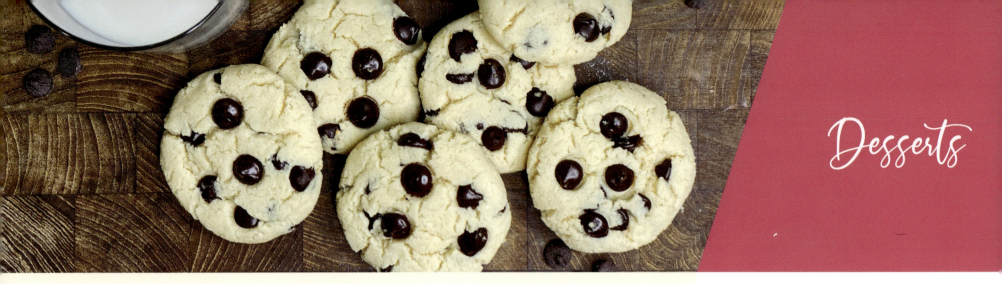

Desserts

Chocolate Chip Protein Cookies

1. Mix the dry ingredients in a large bowl.
2. Add the Greek yogurt and vanilla extract and mash with a spatula or the back of a spoon until a dough begins to form.
3. Gradually add the chocolate chips as you fold the dough. The dough will be thick. Once all the chocolate chips are added, place in the freezer for about 30 minutes to set then preheat the oven to 350°F and line a baking sheet with parchment paper or spray with non-stick spray.
4. Using your hands to roll the dough into a large ball. Divide into 6 pieces and flatten into circles between your palms. Cooking spray on your hands helps prevent sticking.
5. Bake for 10-12 minutes or until the cookies are baked through. They'll be a bit soft on top and will firm after cooling. Enjoy

Ingredients:
- 1/4 cup (28g) Coconut Flour
- 1 scoop (31g) Quest Vanilla Milkshake Protein Powder
- 3 tbsp (27g) Swerve confectioners powdered sugar substitute
- 2 tbsp (24g) Swerve brown sugar substitute
- 1 tbsp (5g) sugar-free vanilla pudding mix
- 1/2 tsp (2g) baking powder
- 1/2 tsp (2g) vanilla extract
- 1/4 tsp (1g) salt
- 1/2 cup (120g) 0% plain Greek yogurt
- 1/4 cup (42g) Lily's semi-sweet chocolate chips

Makes 6 cookies, each:
Cal: 80, F: 2.5g, C: 8g (2g fiber), P: 7.5g

Enjoy in 30 minutes
Prep time: 15   Cook time: 12

Master Your Macros

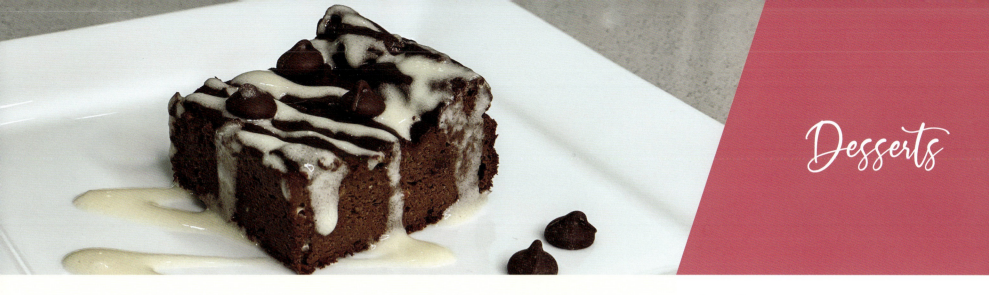

Desserts

Fudge Protein Brownies with Vanilla Icing Drizzle

1. Preheat oven to 350°F and spray 8"×8" baking dish with non-stick spray.
2. Thoroughly mix wet ingredients: applesauce, eggs, brown sugar, and vanilla extract.
3. Add protein powder, brown sugar, cocoa powder, Kodiak cakes mix, baking powder. Mix thoroughly. Fold in the chocolate chips.
4. Pour batter into your dish and bake for 18-22 minutes. The edges will start to harden but the center will still be soft, that's when the brownies are done.
5. Mix icing ingredients while brownies bake.
6. Let brownies cool, slice into 9 squares, drizzle icing. Enjoy!

Ingredients:
- 60g (2 scoops) Quest Chocolate Milkshake protein powder
- 1/2 cup (53g) Kodiak Cakes Buttermilk pancakes mix
- 1/4 cup (20g) unsweetened cocoa powder
- 1/4 cup (37g) Lily's chocolate chips
- 2 large eggs (100g)
- 3/4 cup (180g) unsweetened applesauce
- 1/3 cup (64g) Swerve brown sugar substitute
- 1 tsp (2g) vanilla extract
- 1/4 tsp baking powder

Vanilla Icing Drizzle:
- 15g (1/2 scoop) Quest Vanilla Milkshake protein powder
- 2 tbsp (24g) Swerve confectioners powdered sugar substitute
- 2 tbsp (30mL) unsweetened cashew/almond milk

Makes 9 brownies, each:
Cal: 97, F: 3g, C: 10.8g (3g fiber), P: 10g

Enjoy in 40 minutes
Prep time: **20**   Cook time: **20**

Master Your Macros

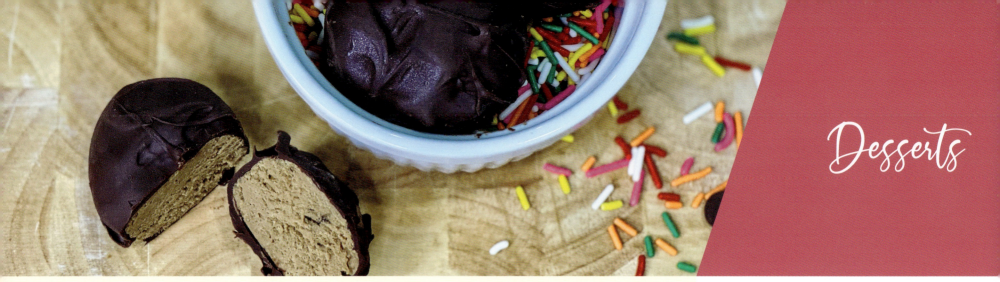

Chocolate Peanut Butter Protein Eggs

1. Microwave peanut butter and syrup for about 15 seconds.
2. Add cream cheese, powdered peanut butter and protein powder to the bowl and knead together until you get a stiff dough.
3. Separate into 5 equal pieces, roll and shape into eggs, set on parchment paper and place in the freezer for one hour.
4. Microwave chocolate chips. You may need 70 grams for dipping but will use around 60g for the eggs.
5. Roll each egg in melted chocolate and place back on parchment paper and refrigerate for 1 hour to allow chocolate to harden. Enjoy!
6. Keep refrigerated for freshness.

Ingredients:
- 2 tbsp (28g) Breanne's Blend Cookie Batter Peanut Butter
- 1/2 cup + 1 tsp (50g) powdered peanut butter
- 1 scoop (31g) Quest Peanut Butter protein powder
- 1 1/2oz. (42g) fat-free cream cheese, softened to room temperature
- 2 tbsp (30mL) sugar-free maple syrup
- 1/3 cup (60g) Lily's chocolate chips

Makes 5 eggs, each:
Cal: 148, F: 7.5 g, C: 16 (5.7g fiber), P: 12.7g

Enjoy in 35 minutes
Prep time: **10**   Cool time: **2 hours**

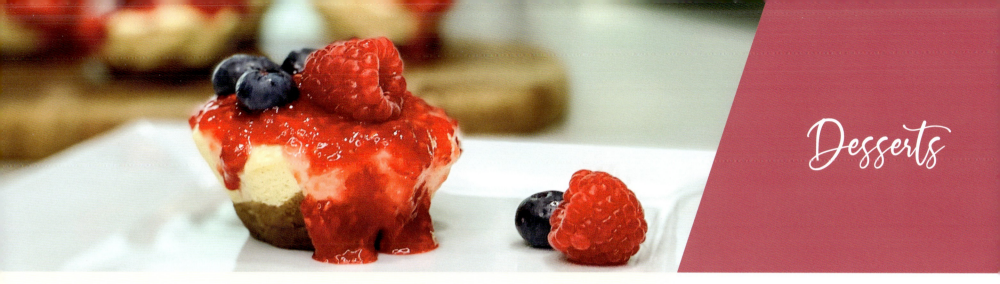

Vanilla Raspberry Protein Mini Cheesecakes

1. Preheat oven to 350°F. Spray 10 spots in a muffin pan with non-stick spray.
2. Crust: Add ingredients to a blender and blend until smooth. Place about 1 tsp mixture in the bottom of each muffin mold and bake in the oven for 5 minutes.
3. Cheesecake: Clean blender and add cream cheese, yogurt and eggs. Process until smooth and creamy. Place in a bowl and mix with remaining ingredients.
4. Spray muffin mold again with non-stick spray and divide the cheesecake filling over the baked crust.
5. Bake for 10-15 minutes. Cheesecake should be a bit jiggly in the center. They will firm in the fridge.
6. Raspberry Drizzle: Add ingredients to a pan over medium heat. Mash raspberries, stir and simmer for a few minutes until sauce thickens.
7. Let cheesecake and raspberry drizzle cool at room temperature then transfer to the fridge for 1-2 hours. Add approx 1 tbsp raspberry drizzle on top of each cheesecake. Enjoy!

Makes 10 cheesecakes, each:
Cal: 118, F: 2g, C: 19.5 (4.5g fiber), P 10g

Enjoy in 2 hour 50 minutes
Prep time: 30 Cook time: 20 Cool time: 2 hours

Graham Cracker Crust:
+ 4 sheets (62g) graham crackers
+ 5 tbsp (88g) unsweetened applesauce
+ 1 tbsp (12g) Swerve brown sugar substitute
+ 1/2 tsp (1g) cinnamon

Cheesecake Filling:
+ 1 package (227g) fat-free cream cheese, softened to room temperature
+ 1 cup (240g) Vanilla Light & Fit Greek Yogurt
+ 2 large eggs (100g)
+ 2 scoops (62g) Quest Vanilla Milkshake protein
+ 1 package (28g) sugar-free cheesecake pudding mix
+ 1 tsp (4g) vanilla extract

Raspberry Drizzle:
+ 1 3/4 cup (220g) fresh raspberries
+ 3 tbsp (27g) Swerve confectioners sugar substitute
+ 1 1/2 tbsp (25g) sugar-free maple syrup
+ 1 1/2 tsp (5g) lemon juice
+ 1/4 tsp (1g) guar gum (thickener)

Master Your Macros

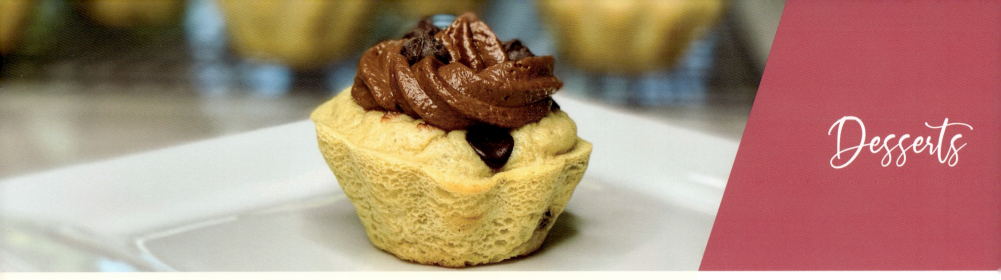

Chocolate & Vanilla Swirl Protein Cupcakes

1. Preheat oven to 350°F and coat 6 cupcake pan mold with non-stick spray.
2. Combine cupcake ingredients in a medium sized bowl and mix until smooth
3. Divide and pour batter into cupcake pan and bake for 15-20 minutes.
4. Mix frosting ingredients while cupcakes are cooking.
5. Let cupcakes cool, top with frosting. Enjoy!

Ingredients:
- 1/2 cup (53g) Kodiak Cake chocolate chip pancake and waffle mix
- 31g (1 scoop) Quest Vanilla Milkshake protein powder
- 2 tbsp (14g) coconut flour
- 1 tsp (4g) vanilla extract
- 1/4 cup (60g) liquid egg whites
- 3/4 cup (180mL) unsweetened almond/cashew milk
- 1/2 tsp (2g) baking powder
- 4 tsp (12g) Swerve granular sugar substitute
- 1 1/2 tbsp (14g) Lily's chocolate chips

Chocolate Protein Frosting:
- 2/3 cup (160g) Light & Fit Greek Vanilla Yogurt
- 15g (1/2 scoop) Quest Chocolate Milkshake protein powder
- 3 tsp (9g) Swerve granular sugar substitute
- 2 tbsp (7g) chocolate sugar-free pudding mix

Makes 6 cupcakes, each:
Cal: 110, F: 2g, C: 12g (2.5g fiber), P: 12g

Enjoy in 35 minutes
Prep time: **15**   Cook time: **20**

Master Your Macros

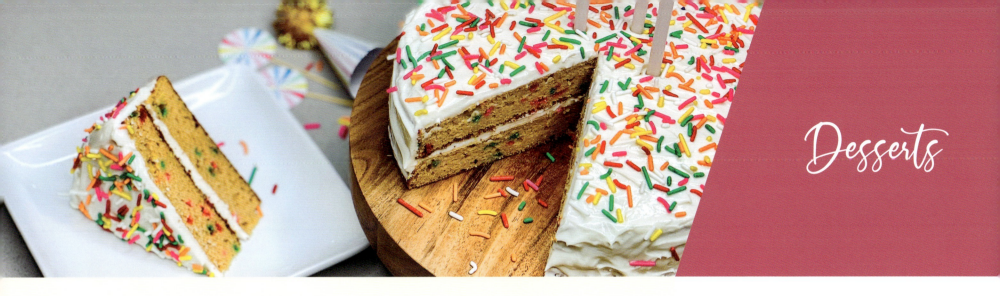

Desserts

Funfetti Protein Cake

1. Preheat oven to 350°F and spray two 8" round cake pans with non-stick cooking spray. Set aside.
2. Mix the dry cake ingredients in a large bowl. Keep sprinkles set aside. Add wet ingredients and whisk together until smooth. Fold 2 tbsp of sprinkles into the batter.
3. Pour half of the batter into each cake pan. Bake for 22-26 minutes or until a toothpick comes out clean. Allow cakes to completely cool before adding the frosting.
4. For the frosting: Blend the cream cheese and vanilla extract until smooth and pour into a medium sized bowl. Add the Greek yogurt and protein powder, mix thoroughly.
5. Frost the top of one cake before placing the second cake on top. Frost the top and sides of both cakes together and top with remaining sprinkles. Enjoy! Refrigerate after serving.

Cake:
- 1 1/2 cups (159g) Kodiak Cakes Buttermilk pancake mix
- 3 scoops (93g) Quest Vanilla Milkshake protein powder
- 1/2 cup (96g) Swerve granular sugar substitute
- 2 tsp (8g) baking powder
- 1 cup (240 mL) unsweetened cashew/almond milk
- 1/2 cup (120g) unsweetened apple sauce
- 1/2 cup (122g) canned pumpkin
- 1 large egg (50g)
- 2 tsp (8g) vanilla extract
- 4 tbsp (40g) sprinkles

Frosting:
- 4oz. (110g) fat-free cream cheese, softened to room temperature
- 1/2 cup (120g) 0% plain Greek yogurt
- 31g (1 scoop) Quest Vanilla Milkshake protein powder
- 2 tbsp (24g) Swerve granular sugar substitute
- 1 tsp (4g) vanilla extract

Makes 8 slices, each:
Cal: 200, F: 3g, C: 32.5g (2.5g fiber), P: 21g

Enjoy in 80 minutes
Prep time: 20 Cook time: 25 Cool time: 35

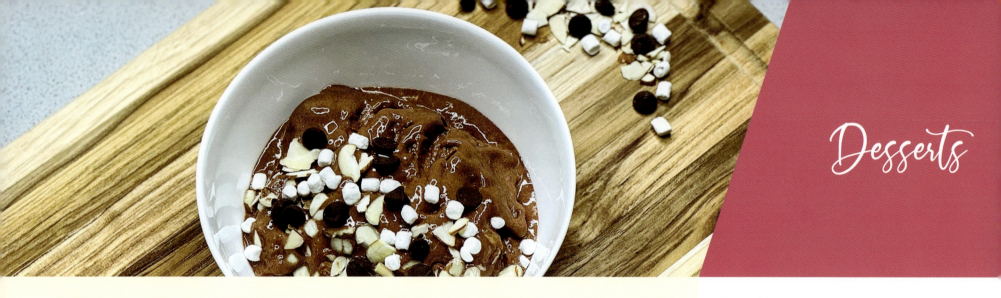

Desserts

Rocky Road Protein Ice Cream

1. Place ice cream ingredients in your blender and blend until smooth.
2. Dish ice cream into a bowl and mix in the toppings. Enjoy!
3. Optional: if you want a firmer ice cream, place the bowl in your freezer for 10-20 minutes.

Ingredients:
- 31g (1 scoop) Quest Chocolate Milkshake protein powder
- 1 cup (240g) ice
- 1/3 cup (80mL) unsweetened cashew/almond milk
- 2 tbsp (10g) unsweetened cocoa powder
- 1 tsp (4g) Swerve granular sugar substitute
- 1/2 tsp (1g) guar gum

Toppings:
- 1 tbsp (7g) chopped almonds
- 1 tbsp (7g) Lily's chocolate chips
- 1 tbsp (3g) mini marshmallows

Makes 1 serving:
Cal: 220, F: 7.5g, C: 24.5g (10g fiber), P: 27.5g

Enjoy in 5 minutes

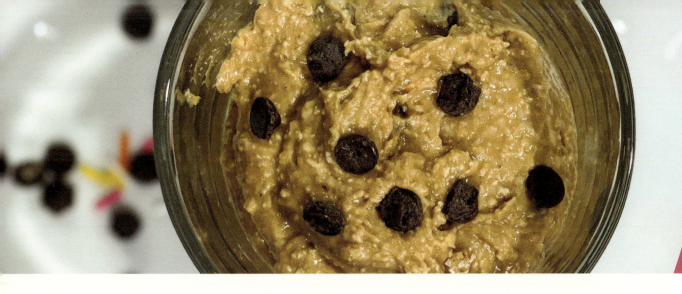

Desserts

Chocolate Chip Protein Cookie Dough

1. Whisk wet and dry ingredients in separate bowls.
2. Slowly add dry ingredients to wet. Use a silicone spatula to mix, continuing to fold it over until it forms a cookie dough.
3. Fold in the chocolate chips, then place in the refrigerator for at least one hour to fully set. It is ready to eat immediately after mixing, but the flavors combine as they sit and create a better cookie dough taste.

Ingredients:
- 31g (1 scoop) Quest Vanilla Milkshake Protein Powder
- 1/4 cup (24g) oat flour
- 2 tbsp (14g) powdered peanut butter
- 1 tbsp (12g) Swerve granular sugar substitute
- 1/2 tsp (2g) salt
- 2 tbsp (30mL) sugar-free maple syrup
- 2 tbsp (30g) 0% plain Greek yogurt
- 1/2 tsp (2g) vanilla extract
- 1 1/2 tbsp (14g) Lily's semi-sweet chocolate chips

Makes 2 servings, each:
Cal: 168, F: 4g, C: 23g (3.5g fiber), P: 18g

Enjoy in 10 minutes

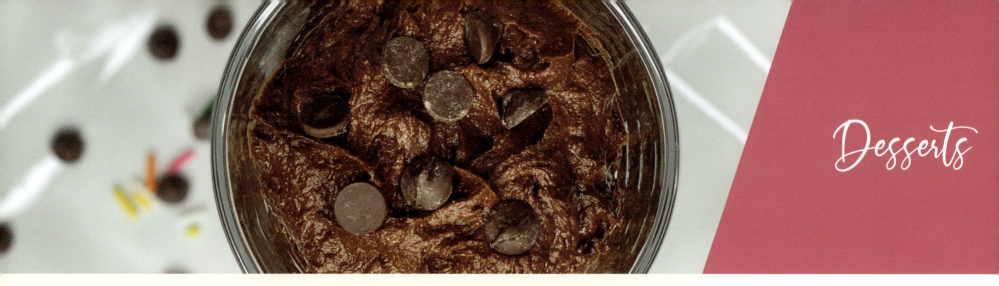

Desserts

Protein Brownie Batter

1. Mix wet and dry ingredients in separate bowls.
2. Slowly add dry ingredients to wet. Use a silicone spatula to mix, continuing to fold it over until it forms a brownie batter.
3. Fold in the chocolate chips, then place in the refrigerator for at least one hour to fully set. It is ready to eat immediately after mixing, but the flavors combine as they sit and create a better brownie batter taste.

Ingredients:
- 31g (1 scoop) Quest Chocolate Milkshake protein powder
- 1 1/2 tbsp (7g) unsweetened cocoa powder
- 1 tbsp (6g) powdered peanut butter
- 2 tbsp (24g) Swerve granular sugar substitute
- 1/4 tsp (1g) salt
- 1/4 cup (61g) canned pumpkin
- 1/2 tsp (2g) vanilla extract
- 2 tbsp (30 mL) sugar-free maple syrup
- 1 1/2 tbsp (14g) Lily's semi-sweet chocolate chips

Makes 2 servings, each:
Cal: 130, F: 3g, C: 17g (7g fiber), P: 14.5g

Enjoy in 10 minutes

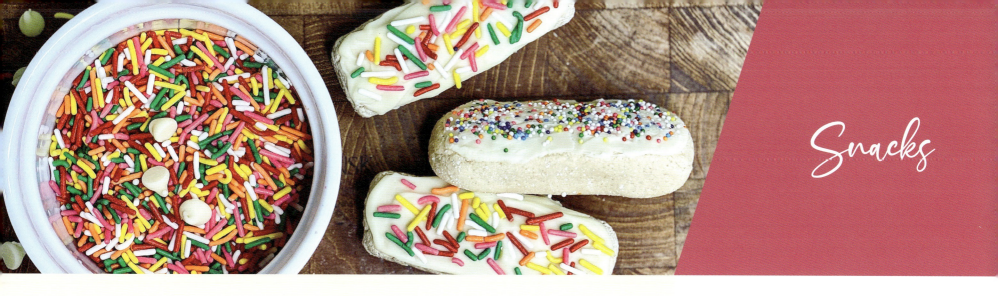

Snacks

Birthday Cake Protein Bars

1. Mix syrup, vanilla extract and almond milk.
2. Add protein powder, sugar, and coconut flour. You want it slightly crumbly.
3. Knead dough together. Once completely mixed, form dough into two bars.
4. Melt white chocolate chips in the microwave and spread half of the melted mixture over the tops of each bar. Top with 1 tsp sprinkles.
5. Keep bars in the fridge for freshness. Enjoy!

Ingredients:

+ 62g (2 scoops) Quest Vanilla Milkshake protein powder
+ 2 tbsp (14g) coconut flour
+ 2 tbsp (30mL) sugar-free maple syrup
+ 1 tbsp (12g) Swerve granular sugar substitute
+ 1 tbsp (15mL) unsweetened almond/cashew milk
+ 1 tsp (4g) vanilla extract
+ 2 tsp (8g) sprinkles
+ 1 1/2 tbsp (14g) Lily's white chocolate chips

Makes 2 bars, each:
Cal: 197, F: 3.5g, C: 23g (7g fiber), P: 25g

Enjoy in 10 minutes

Master Your Macros

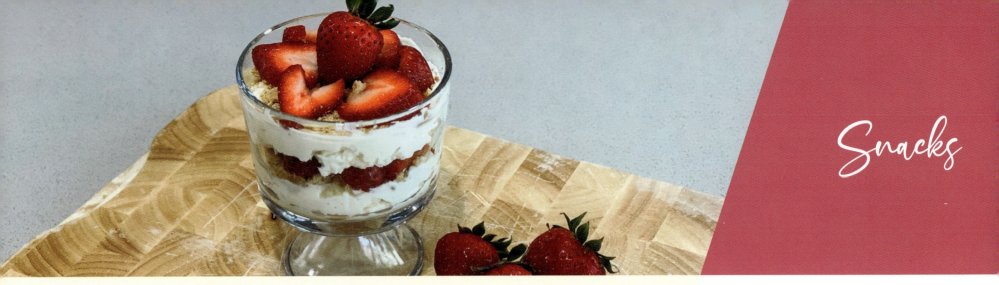

Strawberry Cheesecake Protein Parfait

1. Mix Greek yogurt, pudding mix and protein powder.
2. Dice strawberries and crush graham cracker squares.
3. Place 1/2 yogurt mix in a cup and top with 1/2 graham cracker crumbles and 1/2 diced strawberries.
4. Top with remaining yogurt mix, graham crackers, strawberries and enjoy!

Best served fresh since the graham crackers will soak up some moisture.

Ingredients:
- 3/4 cup (180g) 0% plain Greek yogurt
- 15g (1/2 scoop) Quest Vanilla Milkshake protein powder
- 2 tbsp (7g) cheesecake sugar-free pudding mix
- 1/2 sheet (8g) graham cracker, crushed
- 4 strawberries (48g), diced

Makes 1 serving:
Cal: 240, F: 1g, C: 25g (1g fiber), P: 31g

Enjoy in 5 minutes

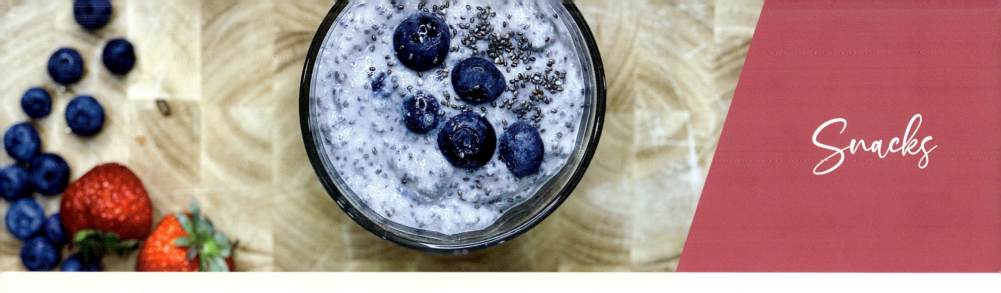

Blueberry Muffin Protein Pudding

1. Mix all ingredients together and allow to stand in the fridge for at least 2 hours to fully combine.

Ingredients:

+ 31g (1 scoop) Quest Vanilla Milkshake protein powder
+ 3/4 cup (180mL) unsweetened cashew/almond milk
+ 2 tbsp (26g) chia seeds
+ 2 tbsp (14g) coconut flour
+ 3 tbsp (45mL) Walden Farms Blueberry Syrup
+ 1/3 cup (50g) fresh blueberries

Eat the whole bowl for breakfast, or split into two 2 servings, each:
Cal: 178, F: 5.5g, C: 14g (8.5g fiber), P: 17g

Enjoy in 125 minutes
Prep time: **5** Cool time: **2 hours**

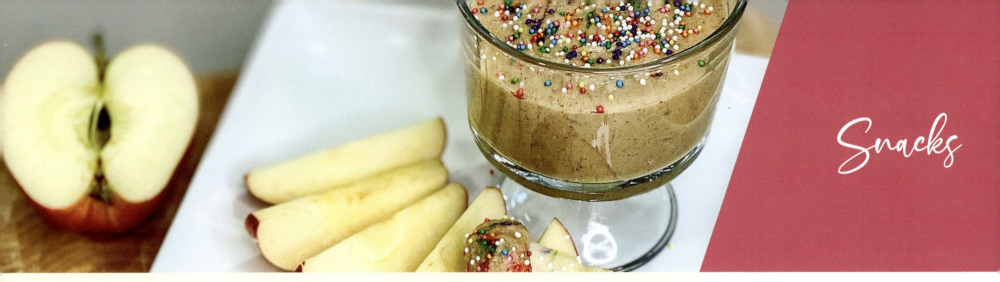

Banana Almond Protein Dip

1. Mash together banana, almond butter and sugar-free maple syrup.
2. Mix in protein powder, coconut flour and salt
3. Top with sprinkles.

Enjoy by the spoonful, or on top sliced apples, graham crackers or animal crackers, etc.

Ingredients:
- 31g (1 scoop) Quest Vanilla Milkshake protein powder
- 1 medium (118g) overripe banana
- 2 tbsp (28g) Confetti Pop Almond Butter by American Dream Nut Butter
- 2 tbsp (14g) coconut flour
- 2 tbsp (30mL) sugar-free maple syrup
- 1/4 tsp (1g) sea salt
- 2 tbsp (24g) sprinkles

Makes 5 servings, each:
Cal: 86, F: 3g, C: 9.5g (2g fiber), P: 6.5g

Enjoy in 10 minutes

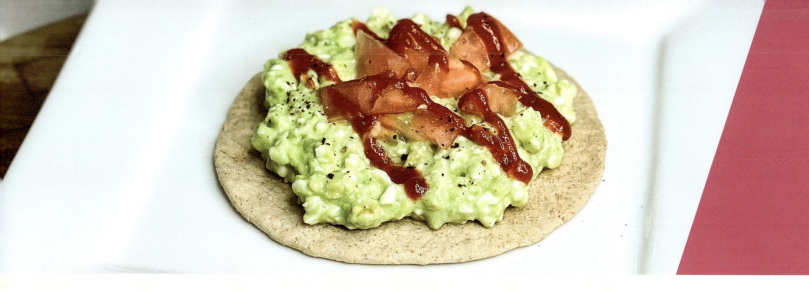

Snacks

Spicy Avocado Protein Toast

Ingredients:
+ 1/4 cup (60g) fat-free cottage cheese
+ 1/4 small avocado (34g)
+ 1 tbsp (15g) sriracha chili hot sauce
+ 1 Mission Carb Balance Street Taco tortilla
+ Diced tomato and black pepper to taste

1. Mash avocado and cottage cheese together with a fork and season with black pepper.
2. Toast tortilla in toaster and top with avocado mixture, diced tomatoes and sriracha hot sauce. Enjoy!

Makes 1 serving:
Cal: 150, F: 6.5g, C: 21.5g (11g fiber), P: 10g

Enjoy in 5 minutes

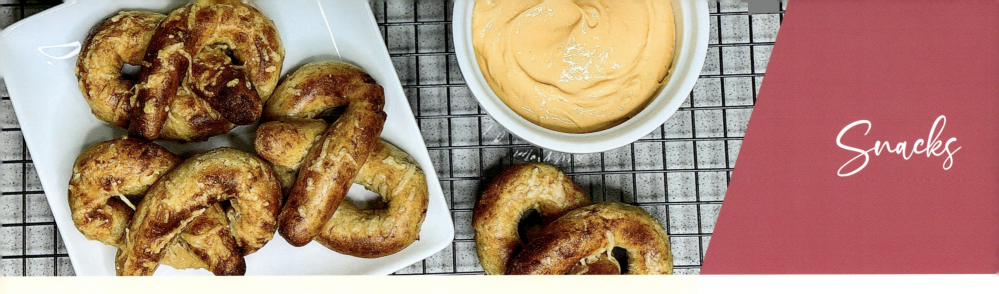

Soft Protein Pretzels with Nacho Cheese Dip

1. Combine Kodiak cakes mix, crushed Quest Chips, Greek yogurt, garlic powder, and baking powder in a bowl and mix until you have a dough ball. Use your hands to knead the dough until all the flour is absorbed.
2. Separate into 4 equal sized pieces (about 90g each) then roll them out with your hands into a tube about 12". Form into the shape of a pretzel. If the dough is too sticky, sprinkle some extra Kodiak Cakes mix on the surface.
3. Brush each formed pretzel with 1/4 egg white and sprinkle 1/2 tbsp parmesan cheese on top.
4. Cook in your air fryer basket at 350°F for 5-8 minutes- depending on how soft you want them.
5. In a microwave safe bowl, mix Greek yogurt and cream cheese and heat for about 30 seconds. Mix in powdered cheese.
6. Let pretzels sit for 5 minutes to cool. Dip in cheese dip and enjoy! Keep refrigerated for freshness.

Snacks

Ingredients:
+ 1 cup + 2 tbsp (120g) Kodiak Cakes Whole Wheat & Honey flapjack and waffle mix
+ 1 bag (32g) Quest Nacho Cheese tortilla style protein chips, crushed into fine pieces
+ 2 tsp (8g) baking powder
+ 1 tsp (4g) garlic powder
+ 2/3 cup (160g) plain 0% Greek yogurt
+ 2 tbsp (10g) grated parmesan cheese
+ 1 tbsp (15g) liquid egg whites

Cheese Dip:
+ 1/3 cup (80g) 0% plain Greek yogurt
+ 1oz. (28g) fat-free cream cheese, softened to room temperature
+ 2 tbsp (14g) Anthony's cheese powder

Makes 4 servings, each:
Cal: 212, F: 3.5g, C: 25.5g (3g fiber), P: 20g

Enjoy in 30 minutes
Prep time: 15   Cook time: 8   Set: 5

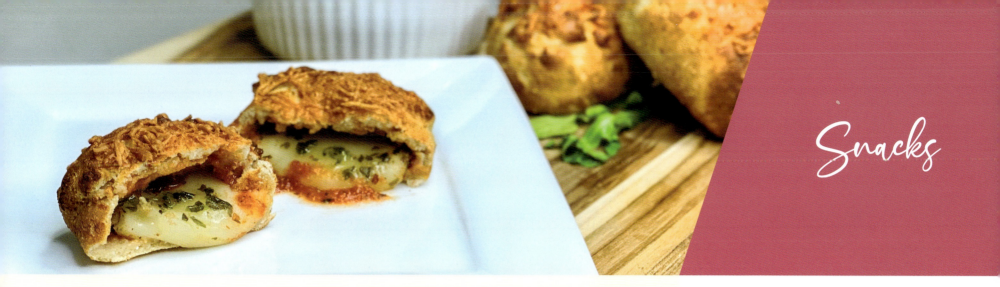

Margherita Pizza Protein Pocket

1. Combine Kodiak Cakes mix, coconut flour, baking soda, and Greek yogurt in a bowl and mix until you have a dough ball. Use your hands to knead the dough until all the flour is absorbed. Divide into three equal pieces, about 63g each.
2. With a rolling pin, flatten each into a thin rectangle.
3. In the center of each rectangle, layer: 1 tsp marinara sauce, 1 babybel cheese, 1/2 tsp basil paste, and top with 1 more tsp marinara sauce.
4. Fold dough over on itself and seal edges to create your pizza pocket.
5. Brush tops of the pockets with liquid egg white and top with 1 tsp parmesan cheese.
6. Cook in your air fryer basket at 350°F for 7-8 minutes. Let it cool until it reaches your preferred temperature.
7. If making ahead of time, heat pizza pockets in microwave for 30-45 seconds, and enjoy!

Ingredients:
+ 1/2 cup (53g) Kodiak cakes buttermilk pancake mix
+ 1/2 cup (120g) 0% Greek yogurt
+ 2 tbsp (14g) coconut flour
+ 2 tsp (8g) baking powder
+ 3 mini Babybel light cheese rounds
+ 2 tbsp (31g) marinara sauce
+ 1 tsp (6g) basil paste
+ 3 tsp (7g) shredded parmesan cheese
+ 1 tbsp liquid egg whites
+ Garlic powder to taste

Makes 3 servings, each:
Cal: 180, F: 5g, C: 17.5g (3.7g fiber), P: 17g

Enjoy in 30 minutes
Prep time: **20**   Cook time: **8**   Set: **2**

Master Your Macros

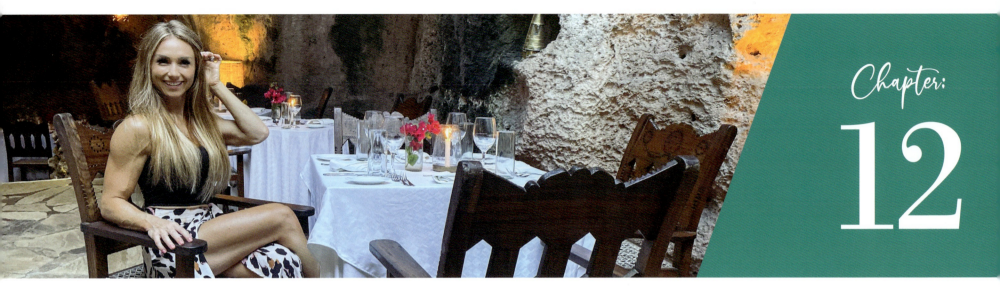

Chapter: 12

Macro-Friendly Restaurant Guide

To make restaurant ordering healthier and easier, I've compiled an extensive list of macro-friendly items from a variety of fast food and chain restaurants. Some menu items may be seasonal, vary by location, and change over time. This isn't a complete list of every great dish these restaurants offer, but it represents a good variety of them. I hand-picked these based on overall calories and protein content. Also, don't be afraid to look at the kid's menu. Kid's portions are typically not oversized, and therefore, nutritional value of some dishes might be a better fit for your health and fitness goals.

Fast Food

Arby's
Roast Beef Classic Sandwich: CAL: 360/ 14F/ 37C/ 23P
Prime-cut Chicken Tenders (3pc): CAL: 360/ 17F/ 28C/ 23P
Double Roast Beef Sandwich: CAL: 510/ 24F/ 38C/ 38P
Turkey Gyro: CAL: 470/ 20F/ 48C/ 25P
Chopped Farmhouse Salad w/ Roast Turkey: CAL: 230/ 3F/ 8C/ 23P

Burger King
Whopper Jr. Sandwich w/o Mayo: CAL: 310 18F /27C /13P
Double Cheeseburger CAL: 390/ 21F/ 27C /23P
Bacon Double Cheeseburger: CAL: 420/ 24F/ 27C/ 25P
Garden Grilled Chicken Salad: CAL 440/ 25F/ 31C/ 25P

Blimpie
Blimpie Best (Rg): CAL: 470/ 5F/ 54C/ 26P
French Dip (Rg): CAL: 430/ 11F/ 53C/ 31P
Grilled Chicken Teriyaki (Rg): CAL: 450/ 10F/ 62C/ 31P
Ham & Swiss (Rg): CAL: 430/ 14F/ 54C/ 25P
Turkey & Avocado (Rg) : CAL: 430/ 11F/ 55C/ 26P
Mediterranean on Ciabatta, Rg: CAL: 400/ 8F/ 49C/ 29P
Pastrami on Ciabatta (Rg): CAL: 400/ 11F/ 45C/ 29P
Roast Beef & Provolone (Rg): CAL: 460/ 14F/ 53C/ 32P

Chick-Fil-A
Egg White Grill: CAL: 300/ 7F/ 31C/ 25P
Chicken Hash Brown Scramble Bowl: CAL: 460 /29 F/ 16C/ 31P
Chicken Egg & Cheese Bagel: CAL: 480 /18 F/ 27P
Grilled Nuggets (12 pc): CAL: 210 / 5 F/ 3C /38P
Grilled Chicken Sandwich: CAL: 310/ 6F/ 36C/ 29P
Grilled Market Salad w/ Grilled Nuggets: CAL: 350/ 14F/ 27C/ 31P
Grilled Chicken Club Sandwich: CAL: 430/ 16F/ 36C/ 37P
Grilled Chicken Cool Wrap: CAL: 350 /14F/ 29C/ 37P
… All of Chick-Fil-A salads seem to be a great option.

Culver's
Buffalo Chicken Tenders (4pc): CAL:460 / 22F/ 32C /34P
Grilled Chicken Sandwich: CAL: 390/ 8F/ 40C /41P
Chicken Cashew Salad w/ Grilled Chicken: CAL:450/ 24F/ 13C/ 46P
Cranberry Bacon Bleu Salad w/ Grilled Chicken: CAL: 360/ 14F/ 14C /44P
Garden Fresco Salad w/ Grilled Chicken: CAL: 350/ 14F/ 15C/ 44P
George's Chili Supreme: CAL: 385/ 20F/ 27C/ 20P

El Pollo Loco
Double Chicken & Avocado Fit Bowl: CAL: 510/ 33F/ 15C/ 41P
Double Chicken & Mango Fit Bowl: CAL: 460/ 26F/ 37P
Double Chicken & Queso Fresco Fit Bowl: CAL: 480/ 27F/ 17C/ 43P
Chicken Tortilla Soup w/o Tortilla Strips (large): CAL: 280/ 10F/ 20C/ 30P
Chicken Double Avocado Salad: CAL: 370/ 14F/ 14C/ 48P
Chicken Avocado Tortilla Wrap: CAL: 480/ 19F/ 46C/ 34P
Chicken Black Bean Bowl: CAL: 460/ 11F/ 57C/ 37P
Chicken Classic Tostada w/o Shell: CAL: 400/ 12F/ 40C/ 32P
Chicken Taco Al Carbon: CAL: 150/ 6F/ 40C/ 10P

Firehouse Subs
Small Chicken Cajun: CAL: 360/ 18F/ 28C/ 23P
Small Club on a Sub: CAL: 390/ 20F/ 32C/ 20P
Small Hero: CAL: 400/ 19F/ 33C/ 24P
Small Hook & Ladder: CAL: 360/ 18F/ 32C/ 18P
Small Cajun Chicken: CAL: 360/ 18F/ 27C/ 23P
Chopped Hook & Ladder Salad: CAL: 260/ 8F/ 21C/ 30P
Firehouse Chopped salad w/ Grilled Chicken: CAL: 380/ 10F/ 27C/ 57P
Firehouse Chopped salad w/ Turkey: CAL: 220/ 7F/ 15C/ 29P
Italian Chopped salad w/ Grilled Chicken: CAL: 410/ 22F/ 14C/ 39P

Hardee's / Carl's Jr.
The 1/3 lb. Lettuce-Wrapped Thickburger: CAL: 420/ 33F/ 8C/ 25P
Big Hamburger: CAL: 480/ 18F/ 56C/ 25P
All-Natural Charbroiled BBQ Chicken Sandwich: CAL:370 49C/ 33P/ 5F/
Hand Breaded Chicken Tenders (5 pc): CAL: 440/ 21F/ 21C/ 41P

Master Your Macros

In-N-Out Burger
Hamburger w/ Protein Style Bun: CAL: 240/ 17F /11C /13P
Hamburger w/ Mustard & Ketchup (instead of spread):
    CAL: 310/ 10F/ 41C/ 16P
Cheeseburger w/ Protein Style Bun: CAL: 330/ 25F/ 11C/ 18P
Cheeseburger w/ Mustard & Ketchup (instead of spread):
    CAL: 400/ 18F/ 41C/ 22P

Jack in the Box
Breakfast Jack: CAL: 280/ 11F/ 30C/ 16P
Ultimate Breakfast Sandwich: CAL: 520/ 10F/ 42C/ 33P
Chicken Fajita Pita made w/ Whole Grain (no salsa):
    CAL: 340/ 12F/ 35C/ 23P
Grilled Chicken Salad w/ Balsamic dressing: CAL: 250/ 9F/ 13C/ 30P
Chicken Sandwich w/ Bacon: CAL: 470/ 25F/ 42C/ 21P
Chicken Club Salad w/ Grilled Chicken: CAL: 370/ 20F/ 11C/ 39P
Southwest Salad w/ Grilled Chicken: CAL: 350/ 15F/ 27C/ 35P

Kentucky Fried Chicken
Original Recipe Chicken Breast: CAL: 390 21F/ 11C/ 39P
Kentucky Grilled Chicken Thigh: CAL: 150/ 9F /0C/ 17P
Kentucky Grilled Chicken Breast: CAL: 210/ 7F/ 0C/ 38P
Kentucky Grilled Chicken Drumstick: CAL: 80/ 4F/ 0C/ 11P
Kentucky Grilled Chicken Wing: CAL: 70/ 3F/ 0C/ 9P
Nashville Hot Kentucky Grilled Chicken Breast: cal: 260/ 3F/ 1C/ 38P
Nashville Hot Kentucky Grilled Chicken Thigh: CAL: 180/ 12F / 0C/ 17P
Crispy Colonel's Chicken Sandwich: CAL: 470/ 24F/ 39C/ 24P
Honey BBQ Sandwich: CAL: 350/ 3.5 F/ 55C/ 24P
BBQ Baked Beans: CAL: 190/ 1F/ 34C/ 11P

McDonald's
Egg McMuffin: CAL: 300/ 12F/ 30C/ 17P
Double Cheeseburger: CAL: 440/ 23F/ 34C/ 25P
Premium Grilled Chicken Sandwich: CAL: 360/ 9F/ 41C/ 27P
Premium Grilled Chicken Ranch BLT Sandwich: CAL: 380/ 10F/ 41C/ 31P
Chipotle BBQ Snack Wrap (Grilled): CAL: 260/ 9F/ 28C/ 18P

Premium Southwest Salad w/ Grilled Chicken: CAL: 320/ 9F/ 30C/ 30P
Premium Bacon Ranch Salad w/ Grilled Chicken: CAL: 260/ 9F/ 12C/ 33P
Premium Caesar Salad w/ Grilled Chicken: CAL: 220/ 6F/ 12C/ 30P

Mission BBQ
Brisket (Lean, 8oz): CAL: 480/ 18F/ 3C/ 73P
Brisket Sandwich (Lean, 6oz.): CAL: 480/ 15F/ 24C/ 59P
Pulled Chicken (Meat Market): CAL: 404/ 18F/ 4C/ 53P
Pulled Chicken Sandwich: CAL: 423/ 19F/ 24C/ 43P
Smoked Salmon: CAL: 373/ 20F/ 0C/ 45P
Turkey Sandwich (6oz): CAL: 418/ 12F/ 23C/ 52P

Panda Express
Grilled Teriyaki Chicken: CAL: 300/ 13F/ 8C/ 36P
Grilled Asian Chicken: CAL: 300 13F/ 8C/ 36P
Teriyaki Chicken: CAL: 340/ 13F/ 14C/ 41P
Asian Chicken: CAL: 340/ 13F/ 14C/ 41P
Black Pepper Angus Steak Entree: CAL: 180/ 7F/ 10C/ 19P
Broccoli Beef: CAL: 150/ 7F/ 13C/ 9P

Popeye's
Chicken Breast: CAL: 380/ 20F/ 16C/ 35P
Chicken Leg: CAL: 160/ 9F/ 5C/ 14P
Blackened Chicken Tenders (3pc): CAL: 170/ 2F/ 2C/ 26P
Blackened Chicken Tenders (5pc): CAL: 283/ 3F/ 3C/ 43P
Loaded Chicken Wrap: CAL: 310/ 12F/ 35C/ 14P

Quizno's
4" Prime Rib XL: CAL: 450/ 19F/ 21C/ 26P
4" Black Angus Steakhouse: CAL: 390/ 13F/ 44C/ 23P
4" Turkey Bacon Guacamole: CAL: 420/ 18F/ 39C/ 24P
4" Mesquite Chicken: CAL: 400/ 17F/ 37C/ 27P
4" Baja Chicken: CAL: 400/ 16F/ 38C/ 26P
4" Honey Mustard Chicken: CAL: 430/ 18F/ 40C/ 27P

Rubios
California Bowl w/ Pan-Seared Shrimp: CAL: 483/ 24F/ 78C/ 23P
California Bowl w/ Grilled Chicken: CAL: 502/ 23F/ 79C/ 34P
Two Grilled Wild Alaska Coho Salmon Taco Plate:
   CAL: 448/ 23F/ 89C/ 33P
Two Blackened Wild Alaska Coho Salmon Taco Plate:
   CAL: 458/ 23F/ 93C / 35P
Two Grilled Regal Springs® Tilapia Taco Plate: CAL: 490/ 25F/ 83C/ 37P
Two Blackened Regal Springs® Tilapia Taco Plate:
   CAL: 500/ 27F/ 89C/ 37P
Two Classic Taco Plate w/ Chicken: CAL: 470/ 29F/ 83C/ 37P
Two Classic Taco Plate w/ Steak: CAL: 440/ 17F/ 83C/ 39P
One Classic Taco Plate w/ Steak: CAL: 308/ 10F/ 63C/ 24P
One Classic Taco Plate w/ Chicken: CAL: 323/ 16F/ 63C/ 23P
One Grilled Gourmet Taco™ w/ Chicken: CAL: 325/ 22F/ 64C/ 29P
Three Rubio's Street Tacos® Plate w/ Chicken: CAL: 392/ 12F/ 73C/ 39P

Sonic
Grilled Chicken Wrap: CAL: 420/ 14F/ 39C/ 31P
Asian Sweet Chili Boneless Wings (6 pc): CAL: 470/ 24F/ 32C/ 30P
Buffalo Boneless Wings (6 pc): CAL: 440/ 28F/ 17C/ 29P
Classic Grilled Chicken Sandwich: CAL: 480/ 22F/ 39C/ 30P
Brioche Breakfast Sandwich Ham: CAL: 470/ 22F/ 40C/ 27P

Subway
6" Black Forest Ham: CAL: 260/ 4F/ 42C/ 18P
6" Chicken Mango Curry: CAL: 330/ 7F/ 43C/ 24P
6" Chicken Tikka: CAL: 290/ 5F/ 39C/ 23P
6" Roast Beef: CAL: 280/ 4.5F/ 40C/ 25P
6" Rotisserie Chicken: CAL: 310/ 6F/ 40C/ 28P
6" Turkey Breast: CAL: 280 3.5F/ 46C/ 18P
6" Black Forest Ham, Egg & Cheese: CAL: 410/ 16F/ 45C/ 24P
6" Steak, Egg and Cheese: CAL: 440/ 18F/ 46C/ 27P
Oven Roasted Chicken Salad: CAL: 130/ 2.5F/ 12C/ 17P
Steak and Cheese Salad: CAL: 210/ 9F/ 15C/ 19P
Roast Beef Salad: CAL: 140/ 3.5F/ 12C/ 19P
...There are plenty more options here!

Starbucks
Reduced-Fat Turkey Bacon & Egg White Sandwich:
   CAL: 230/ 5F/ 28C/ 17P
Spinach, Feta & Egg White Wrap: CAL: 290/ 8F/ 34C/ 20P
Ham, Cheddar & Peppers Sous Vide Egg Bites: CAL: 250/ 16F/ 11C/ 17P
Chipotle Chicken Wrap: CAL: 470/ 19F/ 55C/ 22P
Ham & Swiss Panini: CAL: 480/ 23F/ 41C/ 24P

Taco Bell
Fresco Soft Taco w/ Steak: CAL: 150/ 4F/ 17C/ 10P
Fresco Soft Taco w/ Beef: CAL: 160/ 6F/ 18C/ 8P
Fresco Soft Taco w/ Shredded Chicken: CAL: 150/ 6F/ 16C/ 9P
Power Menu Bowl w/ Chicken: CAL: 470/ 19F/ 50C/ 26P
Power Menu Bowl w/ Steak: CAL: 490/ 20F/ 51C/ 25P
Chicken Soft Taco: CAL: 170/ 8F/ 16C/ 10P

Wendy's
Summer Strawberry Salad (Full): CAL: 410/ 21F/ 17C/ 45P
Apple Pecan Chicken Salad (Full): CAL: 460/ 21F/ 31C/ 39P
Southwest Avocado Chicken Salad (Full): CAL 450/ 26F/ 13C/ 42P
Parmesan Caesar Chicken Salad (Full): CAL: 400/ 21F/ 8C/ 49P
Large Chili: CAL: 330/ 15F/ 30C /22P
Grilled Chicken Sandwich: CAL: 370/ 10F/ 36C/ 34P

Whataburger
Chicken Fajita Taco: CAL: 345/ 12F/ 31C/ 29P
Grilled Chicken Sandwich: CAL: 405/ 11F/ 46C/ 32P
Apple Cranberry Salad w/ Grilled Chicken: CAL: 385/ 12F/ 38C/ 33P
Grilled Chicken Garden Salad: CAL: 290/ 12F/ 12C/ 33P

Zaxby's
The Grilled House Zalad: CAL: 580/ 27F/ 35C/ 52P
The Blackened Blue Zalad: CAL: 530/ 24F/ 34C/ 47P
Grilled Chicken Sandwich: CAL: 480/ 18F/ 38C/ 42P
Boneless Wings (5pc, No sauce): CAL: 330/ 16F/ 22C/ 23P
Traditional Wings (5pc, No sauce): CAL: 380/ 24F/ 3C/ 38P
Chicken Fingers (5pc, No sauce): CAL: 480/ 22F/ 22C/ 49P

Restaurants

Applebee's
Chicken Tortilla Soup: CAL: 190/ 9F/ 18C/ 9P
Top Sirloin (6oz): CAL: 200/ 7F/ 1C/ 34P
Top Sirloin (8oz): CAL: 240/ 10F/ 1C/ 45P
New York Strip (12oz): CAL: 480/ 25F /1C/ 65P
Double Glazed Baby Back Ribs, half rack: CAL: 430/ 32F/ 0C/ 36P
Blackened Cajun Salmon: CAL: 240/ 9F/ 5C/ 35P
Tuscan Garden Chicken Salad: CAL: 350/ 21F/ 16C/ 27P
Grilled Shrimp Skewer: CAL: 110/ 9F/ 1C/ 8P
Kids- Chicken Tenders: CAL: 290/ 16F/ 1C/ 19P
Kids- Chicken Taco: CAL: 230/ 8F/ 19C/ 20P

BJ's Brewhouse
Ahi Poke: CAL: 320/ 10F/ 24C/ 32P
Chicken Lettuce Wraps: CAL 490/ 19F/ 46C/ 31P
BBQ Chicken Deep Dish Pizza- large: CAL: 340/ 10F/ 42C/ 19P
Enlightened Asian Chopped Salad: CAL: 540/ 20F/ 38C/ 45P
Broccoli Cheddar Soup: CAL: 480/ 33F/ 29C/ 19P
Chicken Tortilla Soup: CAL: 280/ 12F/ 30C/ 12P

Bonefish Grill
Cob Imperial: CAL: 480/ 28F/ 7C/ 50P
Cod Piccata: CAL: 400/ 23F/ 13C/ 37P
Filet Mignon (6 oz): CAL: 240/ 9F/ 0C/ 41P
Lily's Chicken: CAL: 470/ 21F/ 9C/ 62P
Ahi Tuna Steak: CAL: 220/ 35F/ 0C/ 46P
Atlantic Salmon (Small): CAL: 330/ 19F/ 0C/ 39P
Georges Bank Scallops & Shrimp: CAL: 250/ 9F/ 4C/ 38P
Rockfish Simply Grilled: CAL: 270/ 7F/ 5C/ 50P
Wood-Grilled Shrimp Skewer: CAL: 160/ 10F/ 3C/ 15P

Buffalo Wild Wings
Traditional Wings (Snack Size w/o Sauce): CAL: 360/ 20F/ 0C/ 44P
Grilled Chicken Buffalitos: CAL: 490/ 20F/ 37C/ 41P
Grilled Chicken Tender Sandwich: CAL: 430/ 10F/ 37C/ 47P
Kids- Naked Tenders: CAL: 100/ 0.5F/ 0C/ 25P
Kids- Hamburger: CAL: 400/ 19F/ 33C/ 23P

California Pizza Kitchen
Dakota Smashed Pea & Barley Soup: CAL: 340/ 0F/ 66C/ 23P
Banh Mi Bowl: CAL: 280/ 33F/ 40C/ 28P
Thai Crunch Salad: CAL: 580/ 36F/ 44C/ 28P
Sonoma Grilled Chicken Flatbread: CAL: 530/ F: 27/ 48C/ 21P
California Cobb (Half w/ Herb Ranch Dressing): CAL: 480/ 37F/ 11C/ 26P
Thai Crunch (Half; w/ Lime Cilantro Dressing): CAL: 590/ 36F/ 44C/ 28P
Shrimp Scampi Zucchini: CAL: 480/ 26F/ 30C/ 27P
Hawaiian Pizza (per slice): CAL: 180/ 4.5F/ 24C/ 11P
The Original BBQ Chicken Pizza (per slice): CAL: 190/ 5F/ 25C/ 11P

Carrabba's
Grilled Asparagus w/ Prosciutto: CAL: 250/ 16F/ 6C/ 22P
Meatballs And Ricotta: CAL: 380/ 22F/ 17C/ 26P
Johnny Rocco Salad: CAL: 540/ 42F/ 11C/ 28P
Mama Mandola's Sicilian Chicken Soup (Bowl): CAL: 200/ 5F/ 22C/ 16P
Sausage & Lentil Soup, Bowl: CAL: 450/ 21F/ 40C/ 24P
Chicken Bryan: CAL: 540/ 27F/ 12C/ 59P
Chicken Marsala: CAL: 440/ 20F/ 5C/ 54P
Pollo Rosa Maria: CAL: 540/ 27F/ 6C/ 65P
Prosciutto Wrapped Pork Tenderloin: CAL: 350/ 17F/ 8C/ 43P
Tuscan-Grilled Chicken: CAL: 290/ 7F/ <1C/ 52P
Veal Marsala: CAL: 410/ 19F/ 10C/ 47P
Mahi Wulfe: CAL: 370/ 16F/ 17C/ 38P
Tilapia Bellimbusto: CAL: 300/ 15F/ 4C/ 45P

The Cheesecake Factory
White Chicken Chili: CAL: 590/ 16F/ 33C/ 79P
White Chicken Chili (ABQ): CAL: 540/ 21F/ 35C/ 58P
Seared Tuna Tataki Salad: CAL: 490/ 29F/ 17C/ 42P
SkinnyLicious® Factory Chopped Salad: CAL: 530/ 30F/ 34C/ 35P
SkinnyLicious® Asian Chicken Salad: CAL: 590/ 24F/ 53C/ 44P
Mexican Tortilla Salad: CAL: 570/ 24F/ 59C/ 30P
SkinnyLicious® Chicken Soft Tacos: CAL: 510/ 15F/ 63C/ 32P
SkinnyLicious® Shrimp Soft Tacos: CAL: 510/ 14F/ 66C/ 31P
Tuscan Chicken: CAL: 590/ 21F/ 19C/ 81P
Lemon-Garlic Shrimp: CAL: 520/ 19F/ 51C/ 33P
SkinnyLicious® Grilled Salmon: CAL: 570/ 34F/ 21C/ 44P
Grilled Steak Medallions: CAL: 440/ 19F/ 24C/ 45P
Grilled Branzino w/ Mediterranean Salsa: CAL: 540/ 28F/ 14C/ 56P
.....There are lots of SkinnyLicious® items to choose from!

Chili's
Grilled Chicken Fajitas: CAL: 510/ 20F/ 22C/ 63P
6oz Sirloin w/ Grilled Avocado: CAL: 330/ 1F6/ 13C/ 38P
Ancho Salmon: CAL: 630/ 30F/ 42C/ 48P
Grilled Chicken Salad: CAL: 440/ 23F/23C/ 37P
Mango-Chile Chicken: CAL: 510/ 20F/ 50C/ 36P
Chicken Enchilada (Bowl): CAL: 410/ 26F/ 24C/ 20P

Cracker Barrel
Egg n' Hashbrown Casserole w/ Sugar Cured Ham:
    CAL: 380/ 24F/ 16C/ 23P
Veggie Casserole: CAL: 370/ 23F/ 22C/ 20P
Homestyle Salad w/ Smokey Southern Grilled Chicken
    CAL: 550/ 30F/ 16C/ 53P
Loaded Baked Potato Bar w/ Bacon Pieces: CAL: 430/ 37F/ 1C/ 27P
Homemade Chicken n' Dumplins: CAL: 300/ 6F/ 35C/ 28P
Grilled Chicken Tenders, each: CAL: 40/ 1F/ 1C/ 4P

Dave & Buster's
Thai Chicken Superfood Chopped Salad: CAL: 411/ 10F/ 43C/ 36P
Fire-Grilled Steak Salad: CAL: 595/ 37F/ 35C/ 34P
Simply Grilled Chicken: CAL: 613/ 38F/ 11C/ 59P
Chicken Tortilla Soup (Bowl): CAL: 227/ 7F/ 24C/ 20P
Tomato Feta Soup (Bowl): CAL: 131/ 7F/ 12C/ 4P

Denny's
Fit Slam: CAL: 450/ 12F/ 59C/ 27P
Fit Fare Veggie Sizzlin' Skillet: CAL: 390/ 16F/ 40C/ 22P
Cobb Salad (No dressing): CAL: 430/ 30F/ 20C/ 22P
BBQ Chicken Tender Sandwich: CAL: 520/ 18F/ 68C/ 24P
Buffalo Chicken Tender Sandwich: CAL: 520/ 26F/ 40C/ 24P
Honey Buttermilk Chicken Tender Sandwich: CAL: 530/ 24F/ 57C/ 25P

Famous Dave's
Hand-Breaded Crispy Chicken Strips: CAL: 380 15F/ 22C/ 40P
Grilled Chicken Breast Sandwich: CAL: 380/ 11F/ 43C/ 31P
Beyond Meat Burger: CAL: 540/ 30F/ 47C/ 26P
BBQ Pulled Chicken Sandwich: CAL: 580/ 23F/ 66C/ 31P
Dave's Award-Winning Chili: CAL: 460/ 28F/ 29C/ 23P

IHOP
Cage-Free Egg White Veggie Omelette: CAL: 370/ 21F/ 26C / 27P
Simple & Fit 2 Egg Breakfast: CAL: 380/ 9F/ 49C/ 27P
Original Buttermilk Pancakes (3pc): CAL: 410/ 17F/ 56C/ 12P
Grilled Tilapia: CAL: CAL: 240/ 10F/ 2C/ 38P
Pork Chops (4 oz): CAL: 250/ 12F/ 0C/ 36P
Sirloin Steak Tips: CAL: 430/ 23F/ 21C/ 38P
T-Bone Steak (10 oz): CAL: 290/ 11F/ 0C/ 49P
The Classic w/ Grilled Chicken: CAL: 520/ 21F/ 42C/ 42P

Joe's Crab Shack
Bucket of Shrimp (18 pc): CAL: 270/ 3.5F/ 10C/ 47P
Caesar Salad w/ Chicken: CAL: 670/ F46/ C18/ P47
Caesar Salad w/ Shrimp: CAL: 530/ F38/ C19/ P28

Bucket of Snow Crab: CAL: 470/ 4F/ 68C/ 42P
Bucket of Queen Crab: CAL: 440/ 3F/ 68C/ 35P
Bucket of Dungeness Crab: CAL: 470/ 3F/ 69C/ 41P
Bucket of King Crab: CAL: 430/ 3F/ 68C/ 33P
Crab Daddy Feast: CAL: 500/ 4F/ 69C/ 47P
Lobster Daddy Feast: CAL: 580/ 4F/ 69C/ 66P
Grilled Malibu Shrimp: CAL: 540/ 19F/ 55C/ 39P
Add on Grilled Shrimp: CAL: 280/ 5F/ 37C/ 20P

Logan's Roadhouse
Chili (Bowl): CAL: 370/ 18F/ 32C/ 18P
Steak & Vegetable Soup (Bowl): CAL: 270/ 14F/ 15C/ 21P
Filet Mignon: CAL: 250/ 6F/ 0C/ 47P
Health Nut Filet Mignon Meal: CAL: 520/ 6F/ 8C/ 2P5
Sirloin (6 oz): CAL: 380/ 21F/ 0C/ 51P
Fall off the Bone Ribs: CAL: 510/ 35F/ 6C/ 41P
Wood-Grilled Chicken Breast, Rice Pilaf, Parmesan Peppercorn:
    CAL: 550/ 32F/ 27C/ 42P
Grilled Shrimp Skewer w/ Rice Pilaf: CAL: 350/ 19F/ 26C/ 17P
Hand Breaded Shrimp w/ Cocktail Sauce: CAL: 470/ 26F/ 29C/ 29P
Coastal Carolina Fried Shrimp w/ Cocktail Sauce:
    CAL: 560/ 44F/ 94C/ 39P
Coastal Carolina Grilled Shrimp w/ Rice Pilaf: CAL: 470/ 23F/ 52C/ 33P
BBQ Grilled Pork Chop: CAL: 380/ 15F/ 9C/ 47P
Healthy & Hearty Grilled Salmon: CAL: 330/ 24F/ 28C/ 38P
Healthy & Hearty Filet (6oz) : CAL: 290/ 17F/ 28C/ 49P
Healthy & Hearty Sirloin (6oz): CAL: 330/ 24F/ 29C/ 39P
Healthy & Hearty Grilled Chicken: CAL: 230/16F/ 31C/ 54P
Cedar Plank Salmon with Marinade: CAL: 460/ 19F/ 14C/ 56P
Tex-Mex Chicken w/ Black Bean Rice: CAL: 530/ 22F/ 41C/ 44P

LongHorn Steakhouse
Seasoned Steakhouse Wings: CAL: 460/ 28F/ 0C/ 53P
Grilled Chicken & Strawberry Salad w/ Vinaigrette:
    CAL: 530/ 19F/ 52C/ 43P
Farm Fresh Field Greens w/ Salmon: CAL: 530/ 29F/ 23C/ 43P
7-Pepper Sirloin Salad: CAL: 490/ 26F/ 22C/ 45P
Hand-Breaded Chicken Tenders (6pc): CAL: 420/ 22F/ 2C/ 30P
LongHorn® Salmon (7oz): CAL: 300/ 16F/ 2C/ 33P
Chicken Fried Chicken: CAL: 400/ 20F/ 21C/ 35P
Flo's Filet (6oz): CAL: 330/ 15F/ 2C/ 37P
Flo's Filet (9oz): CAL: 450/ 19F/ 3C/ 56P
Renegade Sirloin (6oz): CAL: 320/ 15F/ 2C/ 36P
Renegade Sirloin (8oz): CAL: 390/ 16F/ 2C/ 51P
Nolan Ryan Beef Chicken Fried Steak: CAL: 450/ 26F/ 24C/ 30P
Renegade Sirloin (6oz) w/ Redrock Grilled Shrimp:
    CAL: 480/ 18F/ 4C/ 66P
Hand-Breaded Chicken Tenders (6pc): CAL: 420/ 22F/ 19C/ 36P
LongHorn® Salmon (7oz): CAL: 300/ 16F/ 2C/ 33P
Redrock Grilled Shrimp (8pc): CAL: 160/ 3F/ 2C/ 30P

Lucille's BBQ
BBQ Tri Tip (7oz): CAL: 418/ 19F/ 19C/ 42P
Wedge Salad (add on): CAL: 290/ 20F/ 10C/ 20P
BBQ Tri Tip (Lunch): CAL: 368/ 16F/ 18C/ 35P
Apple Pecan Chicken Salad (Half): CAL: 595/ 34F/ 33C/ 40P
Kids- Aunt Mari's Chicken Supper: CAL: 270/ 0F/ 30C/ 30P
Kids- Grandpa Joe's Tri Tip Supper: CAL: 150/ 10F/ 0C/ 20P
Kids- Homemade Macaroni-n-Cheese: CAL: 409/ 20F/ 39C/ 18P
Kids- Lil' Chicken Fingers: CAL: 360/ 20F/ 20C/ 20P
Kids- Lucy's Cheeseburger: CAL: 531/ 11F/ 2C/ 30P

Maggiano's Little Italy
Italian Wedding Bowl Soup: CAL: 390/ 21F/ 34C/ 18P
Shrimp Fra Diavolo (Lt): CAL: 410/ 13F/ 38C/ 36P
Steak & Veal Oscar Style: CAL: 530/ 40F/ 15C/ 28P
Kids- Cheese Ravioli: CAL:430/ 23F/ 39C/ 21P
Kids- Grilled Chicken: CAL: 450/ 27F/ 28C/ 30P

McAlister's Deli

Pecanberry Salad: CAL: 350/ 12F/ 30C/ 34P
Traditional Chili (Bowl): CAL: 370/ 17F/ 33C/ 26P
Grilled Chicken Salad: CAL: 500/ 25F/ 21C/ 50P
Italian Chopped Salad: CAL: 570/ 42F/ 16C/ 33P
McAlister's Chef Salad: CAL: 480/ 26F/ 21C/ 40P
Savannah Chopped Salad: CAL: 480/ 16F/ 43C/ 40P
Corned Beef Sandwich: CAL: 550/ 13F/ 70C/ 37P
Grilled Chicken Sandwich: CAL: 510/ 6F/ 71C/ 42P
Ham Sandwich: CAL: 520/ 10F/ 71C/ 33P
Pastrami Sandwich: CAL: 540/ 13F/ 70C/ 37P
Roast Beef Sandwich: CAL: 520/ 9F/ 69C/ 37P
Turkey Sandwich: CAL: 470/ 6F/ 70C/ 31P
French Dip Sandwich: CAL: 530/ 15F/ 43C/ 49P

O'Charley's

Peach Chutney Chicken (No side): CAL: 470/ 8F/ 69C/ 31P
Honey-Drizzled Southern Fried Chicken: CAL: 430/ 25F/ 18C/ 30P
Grilled Top Sirloin (6 oz, No Side): CAL: 270/ 18F/ 0C/ 25P
Cedar-Planked Salmon (No Side): CAL: 470/ 28F/ 2C/ 50P
Fresh Atlantic Grilled Salmon, Blackened (6 oz, No Side): CAL: 340/ 21F/ 3C/ 34P
Fresh Atlantic Grilled Salmon, Bourbon (6 oz, No Side): CAL: 430/ 21F/ 29C/ 34P
Fresh Atlantic Grilled Salmon, Chipotle (6 oz, No Side): CAL: 460/ 21F/ 32C/ 37P
Chicken Tortilla Soup: CAL: 190/ 7F/ 20C/ 13P
Kids- Chicken Tenders (No Side): CAL: 340/ 16F/ 12C/ 29P
Kids- Grilled Chicken Breast (No Side): CAL: 160/ 5F/ 3C/ 27P
Kids- Grilled Chicken Salad (No Side): CAL: 240/ 9F/ 19C/ 23P

Olive Garden

Chicken & Gnocchi Soup: CAL: 230/ 12F/ 22C/ 11P
Minestrone Soup: CAL: 110/ 1F/ 17C/ 5P
Cheese Ravioli w/ Marinara Sauce (Lunch): CAL: 450/ 22F/ 40C/ 24P
Cheese Ravioli w/ Meat Sauce (Lunch): CAL: 500/ 26F/ 39C/ 29P
Grilled Chicken Margherita (lunch): CAL: 350/ 18F/ 13C/ 36P
Shrimp Scampi (Lunch): CAL: 480/ 19F/ 53C/ 20P
Grilled Chicken Margherita (dinner): CAL: 520/ 24F/ 15C/ 64P
Herb-Grilled Salmon (Dinner): CAL: 460/ 29F/ 8C/ 45P
Herb-Grilled Salmon Coho (Dinner): CAL: 360/ 15F/ 8C/ 50P
Shrimp Scampi (Dinner): CAL: 510 180/ 7F/ 54C/ 29P
Kids- Grilled Chicken: CAL: 150/ 5F/ 1C/ 27P
Kids- Shrimp: CAL: 30/ 0F/ 0C/ 7P
Kids- Chicken Fingers & Pasta: CAL: 400/ 16F/ 42C/ 24P

Outback Steakhouse

Seared Peppered Ahi, Large: CAL: 430/ 26F/ 17C/ 31P
Wood-Fire Grilled Shrimp on the Barbie: CAL: 540/ 25F/ 44C/ 34P
Asian Salad with Chicken (No Dressing): CAL: 360/ 7F/ 18C/ 53P
Asian Salad with Ahi Tuna (No Dressing):CAL: 240/ 8F/ 12C/ 32P
Outback Center-Cut Sirloin (6oz): CAL: 210/ 7F/ 0C/ 38P
Victoria's Filet Mignon (6oz): CAL: 240/ 9F/ 0C/ 40P
Sirloin (6 oz) & Grilled Shrimp on the Barbie :CAL: 370/ 15F/ 4C/ 52P
Lobster Tail Grilled (5oz): CAL: 420/ 33F/ 1C/ 2P7
Lobster Tail Steamed (5oz): CAL: 340/ 24F/ 1C/ 27P
Chicken Tortilla Soup, Cup: CAL: 170/ 9F/ 13C/ 9P
Bacon Bourbon Salmon (7 oz): CAL: 480/ 32F/ 3C/ 45P
Grilled Alaskan Halibut: CAL: 310/ 7F/ 3C/ 55P
Hand-Breaded Shrimp: CAL: 470/ 20F/ 43C/ 31P
Lobster & Mushroom Topped Mahi: CAL: 410/ 17F/ 8C/ 59P
Perfectly Grilled Salmon (7oz): CAL: 380/ 25F/ 1C/ 38P
Simply Grilled Mahi: CAL: 220/ 3.5F/ 1C/ 47P
Simply Grilled Tilapia: CAL: 250/ 8F/ 2C/ 42P
Tilapia with Pure Lump Crab Meat: CAL: 510/ 27F/ 7C/ 58P
Alice Springs Chicken (5oz): CAL: 440/ 27F/ 9C/ 42P

Panera Bread

Bacon, Egg & Cheese on Brioche: CAL: 450/ 25F/ 33C/ 24P
Bacon, Egg & Cheese on Artisan Ciabatta: CAL: 440/ 19F/ 40C/ 25P
Bacon, Egg & Tomato Wrap: CAL: 430/ 23F/ 32C/ 28P
Asian Sesame Salad with Chicken (Whole): CAL: 430/ 23F/ 29C/ 31P
BBQ Chicken Salad (Whole): CAL: 520/ 4F/ 44C/ 33P
Caesar Salad with Chicken (Whole): CAL: 460/ 28F/ 21C/ 34P
Green Goddess Cobb Salad with Chicken (Whole):
    CAL: 530/ 30F/ 27C/ 42P
Spicy Thai Salad with Chicken (Whole):
    CAL: 490/ 21F/ 43C/ 37P
Strawberry Poppyseed Salad with Chicken (Whole):
    CAL: 360/ 15F/ 34C/ 28P
Smokehouse BBQ Chicken on White Miche (½ Sandwich):
    CAL: 380 130 15F/ 41C/ 21P
Steak & White Cheddar on Artisan Ciabatta (½ Panini):
    CAL: 430/ 18F/ 43C/ 24P

P.F. Chang's

Edamame with Kosher Salt: CAL: 400/ 17F/ 25C/ 37P
Handmade Shrimp Dumplings Steamed (6pc): CAL: 290/ 6F/ 31C/ 26P
Hot & Sour Soup Bowl: CAL: 470/ 12F/ 63C/ 26P
Wonton Soup Bowl: CAL: 570/ 17F/ 53C/ 49P
Ginger Chicken with Broccoli: CAL: 480/ 12F/ 41C/ 57P
Pepper Steak Steamed: CAL: 440/ 21F/ 28C/ 33P
Buddha's Feast Steamed: CAL: 260/ 4F/ 32C/ 25
Shrimp w/ Lobster Sauce Steamed: CAL: 370/ 18F/ 14C/ 31P
Mongolian Beef Bowl: CAL: 490/ 28F/ 89C/ 45P
Ginger Chicken with Broccoli Bowl: CAL: 330/ 9F/ 31C/ 32P
Beef & Broccoli Bowl: CAL: 370/ 19F/ 29C/ 22P

Red Lobster

Lighthouse Garlic-Grilled Shrimp: CAL: 390/ 16F/ 34C/ 30P
Lighthouse Maple-Glazed Chicken: CAL: 370/ 5F/ 53C/ 30P
Lighthouse Rock Lobster Tail: CAL: 400/ 9F/ 35C/ 45P
Lighthouse Snow Crab Legs: CAL: 430/ 34F/ 8C/ 23P
Lighthouse Wood-Grilled Peppercorn Sirloin & Shrimp:
    CAL: 520/ 18F/ 36C/ 54P
Live Maine Lobster (Steamed) 530 310 35 21 0 430 1130 0 0 0 54
Live Maine Lobster (Roasted & Stuffed): CAL: 440/ 10F/ 21C/ 65P
Maple-Glazed Chicken: CAL: 450/ 7F/ 46C/ 52P
Wood-Grilled Peppercorn Sirloin: CAL: 430/ 18F/ 27C/ 40P
Wood-Grilled Peppercorn Sirloin & Shrimp: CAL: 540/ 24F/ 28C/ 52P
Seafood-Stuffed Flounder: CAL: 230/ 13F/ 8C/ 20P
Wood-Grilled Fresh Tilapia: CAL: 210/ 6F/ 0C/ 41P
Wood-Grilled Sirloin: CAL: 240/ 9F/ 3C/ 36P
Canadian Walleye Blackened: CAL: 440/ 9F/ 3C/ 81P
Canadian Walleye Broiled: CAL: 420/ 1.5F/ 0C/ 81P
Arctic Char: CAL: 350/ 16F/ 0C/ 41P
Cod: CAL: 200/ 3F/ 0C/ 40P
Fresh Flounder: CAL: 200/ 4.5F/ 0C/ 35P
Grouper: CAL: 210/ 3.5F/ 0C/ 42P
Haddock: CAL: 170/ 2.5F/ 0C/ 34P
Halibut: CAL: 200/ 4F/ 0C/ 38P
Lake Whitefish: CAL: 310/ 14F/ 0C/ 42P
Opah: CAL: 210/ 3F/ 0C/ 42P
…. and MANY MORE lean fish options!

Red Robin

Veggie Vegan Burger w/ Steamed Broccoli: CAL: 260/ 11F/ 34C/ 13P
Keep It Simple Beef Burger: CAL: 530/ 24F/ 44C/ 34P
The Wedgie™ Burger: CAL: 550/ 35F/ 19C/ 39P
Red's Tavern Double®: CAL: 590/ 36F/ 32C/ 37P
Ensenada Chicken™ Platter (One Breast): CAL: 280/ 12F/ 16C/ 31P
Chicken Tortilla Soup Bowl: CAL: 390/ 19F/ 37C/ 20P
Red's Chili Chili™ Bowl: CAL: 430/ 18F/ 36C/ 28P
Simply Grilled Chicken Salad: CAL: 280/ 8F/ 20C/ 35P

Kids- Red's Cheeseburger Beef: CAL: 350/ 17F/ 30C/ 22P
Kids- Red's Cheeseburger Chicken: CAL: 340/ 9F/ 30C/ 37P
Kids- Red's Cheeseburger Turkey: CAL 450/ 22F/ 31C/ 31P
Kids- Grilled Chicken Dip'Ns: CAL: 120/ 1F/ 0C/ 27P

Romano's Macaroni Grill
Italian Chopped Salad: CAL: 490/ 34F/ 20C/ 27P
Bibb + Bleu Salad w/ Chicken: CAL: 680/ 43F/ 18C/ 61P
Bibb + Bleu w/ Shrimp: CAL: 590/ 43F/ 18C/ 36P
Pollo Caprese: CAL: 560/ 22F/ 40C/ 50P
Chicken Parmesan Sandwich Mix + Match: CAL: 380/ 30F/ 42C/ 25P

Ruby Tuesday
Plain Grilled Petite Sirloin: CAL: 375/ 15F/ 3C/ 55P
Plain Grilled Top Sirloin: CAL: 290/ 12F/ 0C/ 46P
House Sirloin: CAL: 298/ 15F/ 2C/ 39P
Petite Sirloin: CAL: 284/ 19F/ 4C/ 29P
Veggie Burger: CAL: 550/ 21F/ 64C/ 28P
Turkey Burger Wrap: CAL: 590/ 27F/ 46C/ 49P
Grilled Chicken Salad: CAL: 362/ 11F/ 20C/ 18P
Grilled Chicken Wrap: CAL: 443/ 16F/ 40C/ 29P
Chicken Florentine: CAL: 378/ 14F/ 9C/ 54P
Chicken Strips - Traditional : CAL: 177/ 9F/ 12C/ 12P
Chicken Strips - Barbecue: CAL: 203/ 9F/ 18C/ 13P
Chicken Tortilla Soup: CAL: 194/ 8F/ 17C/ 15P
Grilled Salmon: CAL: 330/ 18F/ 0C/ 42P
Blackened Tilapia: CAL: 200/ 7F/ 0C/ 32P
Trout Almondine (Fit Trim, Small Plate): CAL: 550/ 37F/ 28C/ 33P
Creole Catch: CAL: 240/ 10F/ 0C/ 38P
Herb Crusted Tilapia: CAL: 402/ 24F/ 9C/ 36P

Texas Roadhouse
Boneless Buffalo Wings w/ Hot Sauce: CAL: 430/ 25F/ 21C/ 29P
Boneless Buffalo Wings w/ Mild Sauce: CAL: 380/ 21F/ 19C/ 30P
Texas Red Chili (Cup): CAL: 290/ 6F/ 16C/ 21P
Texas Red Chili (Bowl): CAL: 490/ 27F/ 27C/ 35P
Dallas Filet (6 oz): CAL: 270/ 10F/ 2C/ 45P
New York/Kansas City Strip (8 oz): CAL: 420/ 22F/ 1C/ 57P
USDA Choice Sirloin (6 oz) : CAL: 250/ 6F/ 3C/ 46P
Chicken Critters® with Sirloin (6 oz): CAL: 520/ 18F/ 19C/ 72P
Sirloin 8 oz with Grilled Shrimp: CAL: 570/ 16F/ 30C/ 78P
California Grilled Chicken: CAL: 490/ 22F/ 23C/ 55P
Chicken Critters®: CAL: 480/ 21F/ 26C/ 45P
Grilled Pork Chops (Single): CAL: 290/ 12F/ 4C/ 41P
Grilled Salmon (5 oz): CAL: 320/ 24F/ 1G/ 27P
Kids- Grilled Chicken: CAL: 160/ 2.5F/ 1C/ 34P
Kids- Jr. Chicken Tenders: CAL: 360/ 6F/ 24C/ 31P
Kids- Lil' Dillo Steak Bites: CAL: 170/ 4F/ 1C/ 31P

T.G.I. Friday's
BBQ Chicken Salad w/ BBQ Ranch (Lunch): CAL: 560/ 32F/ 43C/ 29P
Million Dollar Cobb Salad w/ Grilled Chicken w/ Ranch (Lunch):
CAL: 520/ 37F/ 13C/ 34P
Bacon Cheeseburger (Green Style, No Side): CAL: 580/ 43F/ 12C/ 35P
BBQ Chicken Wrap: CAL: 580/ 23F/ 61C/ 32P
Grilled Chicken Caesar Wrap: CAL: 580/ 33F/ 43C/ 28P
Soup, Chili: CAL: 340/ 20F/ 18C/ 20P
Bacon Ranch Chicken Sandwich (No side): CAL: 280/ 11F/ 47C/ 55P

Wood Ranch BBQ

Asian Chicken Salad (no dressing) CAL: 536/ 25F/ 45C/ 36P
Baby Back Ribs w/o Sauce (5 bones): CAL: 338/ 25F/ 0C/ 29P
Boneless Chicken Breast w/ Sauce (5 oz): CAL: 185/ 3F/ 7.5C/ 28.5P
Brisket (Lunch, 7 oz): CAL: 308/ 15F/ 0C/ 42P
Balsamic Shrimp w/ Rice: CAL: 405/ 7F/ 60C/ 61P
Chophouse Filet (6 oz): CAL: 285/ 14F/ 2C/ 35P
Prime Top Sirloin (8 oz): CAL: 370/ 17F/ 1C/ 48P
Salmon (Blackened or Grilled, 9 oz): CAL: 486/ 24F/ 1C/ 58P
Trout (Blackened or Grilled, 8-9 oz); CAL: 346/ 17F/ 0C/ 45P
Kid's Baby Back Ribs (5 bones): 338/ 25F/ 0C/ 29P
Kid's- Beef Rib (1 bone): CAL: 248/ 12F/ 17C/ 21P
Kid's- Grilled Chicken Breast (5 oz): CAL: 305/ 3F/ 34C/ 29P
Kid's- Salmon (4 oz): CAL: 243/ 12F/ 0C/ 29P

Yard House

Blackened Shrimp Taco (each): CAL: 170/ 7F/ 16C/ 12P
Kale Caesar w/ Ahi (Small): CAL: 580/ 40F/ 20C/ 33P
Roasted Halibut: CAL: 500/ 20F/ 30C/ 49P
Shrimp Zoodle Bowl: CAL: 470/ 31F/ 19C/ 28P
Steak Bowl: CAL: 530/ 19F/ 48C/ 42P
Chicken Bowl: CAL: 480/ 15F/ 48C/ 42P
Shrimp Bowl: CAL: 440/ 13F/ 49C/ 36P
Classic Sliders (2pc, Lunch): CAL: 490/ 24F/ 41C/ 28P
Artic Char: CAL: 380/ 17F/ 0C/ 53P
Barramundi: CAL: 260/ 5F/ 0C/ 50P
Corvina: CAL: 300 / 12F / 0C/ 44P
Grouper: CAL: 240/ 2.5F/ 0C/ 51P
Mahi Mahi: CAL: 230/ 2F/ 0C/ 49P
Kids- BBQ Chicken: CAL: 260/ 5F/ 20C/ 34P
Kids- Chicken Teriyaki: CAL: 290/ 4.5F/ 28C/ 35P

Acknowledgments

Writing this guide was harder than I thought when I had this crazy idea a year ago, however, the journey has been more rewarding than I could have ever imagined. None of this would be possible without my loving husband, Joel. Thank you for your relentless encouragement to pursue my passion. You set the example daily for what's possible with hard work and determination. You are my best friend, favorite recipe critic, and my rock.

I'm eternally grateful to my dear friend Marisa. Your words of wisdom ignited my fire to write this guide. And not only are you my personal stylist but the magician behind the lens. This guide wouldn't be the same without your eye for capturing my best side.

I'm forever grateful to Daniel and Melinda for their keen insight and for helping bring my words to life.

And to my family. Mom: thank you for setting the example of what a strong woman is capable of. I wouldn't be who I am today without your love and guidance over the last four decades. To my sister: Tallia, my aunts: Linda and 'Mumsie,' my father: Borre (RIP), and step-father: Curtis (RIP). We're a small, strong, and mighty family. I love (and miss) you all so much!

Finally, to you, the reader, and everyone who took a chance on my tips and advice when you felt overwhelmed on your health and fitness journey. I completely understand your frustrations and wrote this guide for you! I'm excited for you to learn, be empowered over your nutrition, and crush your goals.

References

1. Mcmurray RG, Soares J, Caspersen CJ, Mccurdy T. Examining Variations of Resting Metabolic Rate of Adults [Internet]. Medicine & Science in Sports & Exercise2014;46:1352–8. Available from: http://dx.doi.org/10.1249/mss.0000000000000232
2. Astrup A. Carbohydrates as macronutrients in relation to protein and fat for body weight control [Internet]. International Journal of Obesity2006;30:S4–9. Available from: http://dx.doi.org/10.1038/sj.ijo.0803485
3. pubmeddev, Hermsdorff HH E al. [Macronutrient profile affects diet-induced thermogenesis and energy intake]. - PubMed - NCBI [Internet]. [cited 2020 Feb 15];Available from: https://www.ncbi.nlm.nih.gov/pubmed/17824197
4. Sadie B. Barr JCW. Postprandial energy expenditure in whole-food and processed-food meals: implications for daily energy expenditure. Food Nutr. Res. [Internet] 2010 [cited 2020 Feb 10];54. Available from: https://www.ncbi.nlm.nih.gov/pmc/articles/PMC2897733/
5. Thermogenic Effect of Food [Internet]. probefitblog2017 [cited 2020 Feb 10];Available from: https://probefit.com/nutrition/thermogenic-effect-of-food/
6. von Loeffelholz C, Birkenfeld A. The Role of Non-exercise Activity Thermogenesis in Human Obesity. In: Endotext [Internet]. MDText.com, Inc.; 2018.
7. Villablanca PA, Alegria JR, Mookadam F, Holmes DR Jr, Wright RS, Levine JA. Nonexercise activity thermogenesis in obesity management. Mayo Clin. Proc. 2015;90:509–19.
8. Feng RN, Niu YC, Sun XW, Li Q, Zhao C, Wang C, et al. Histidine supplementation improves insulin resistance through suppressed inflammation in obese women with the metabolic syndrome: a randomised controlled trial. Diabetologia 2013;56:985–94.
9. Dietary threonine deficiency depressed the disease resistance, immune and physical barriers in the gills of juvenile grass carp (Ctenopharyngodon idella) under infection of Flavobacterium columnare. Fish Shellfish Immunol. 2018;72:161–73.
10. Mohajeri MH, Wittwer J, Vargas K, Hogan E, Holmes A, Rogers PJ, et al. Chronic treatment with a tryptophan-rich protein hydrolysate improves emotional processing, mental energy levels and reaction time in middle-aged women. Br. J. Nutr. 2015;113:350–65.
11. Berry J. Essential amino acids: Definition, benefits, and foods [Internet]. Medical News Today2019 [cited 2020 Jul 26];Available from: https://www.medicalnewstoday.com/articles/324229
12. Layman DK, Boileau RA, Erickson DJ, Painter JE, Shiue H, Sather C, et al. A Reduced Ratio of Dietary Carbohydrate to Protein Improves Body Composition and Blood Lipid Profiles during Weight Loss in Adult Women. J. Nutr. 2003;133:411–7.

13. pubmeddev, Paddon-Jones D E al. Protein, weight management, and satiety. - PubMed - NCBI [Internet]. [cited 2020 Feb 12]; Available from: https://www.ncbi.nlm.nih.gov/pubmed/18469287

14. White BD, He B, Dean RG, Martin RJ. Low protein diets increase neuropeptide Y gene expression in the basomedial hypothalamus of rats. J. Nutr. [Internet] 1994 [cited 2020 Aug 9];124. Available from: https://pubmed.ncbi.nlm.nih.gov/8064364/

15. Gannon MC, Nuttall FQ. Effect of a high-protein diet on ghrelin, growth hormone, and insulin-like growth factor-I and binding proteins 1 and 3 in subjects with type 2 diabetes mellitus. Metabolism [Internet] 2011 [cited 2020 Aug 9];60. Available from: https://pubmed.ncbi.nlm.nih.gov/21406307/

16. Lejeune MP, Westerterp KR, Adam TC, Luscombe-Marsh ND, Westerterp-Plantenga MS. Ghrelin and glucagon-like peptide 1 concentrations, 24-h satiety, and energy and substrate metabolism during a high-protein diet and measured in a respiration chamber. Am. J. Clin. Nutr. [Internet] 2006 [cited 2020 Aug 9];83. Available from: https://pubmed.ncbi.nlm.nih.gov/16400055/

17. Lomenick JP, Melguizo MS, Mitchell SL, Summar ML, Anderson JW. Effects of meals high in carbohydrate, protein, and fat on ghrelin and peptide YY secretion in prepubertal children. J. Clin. Endocrinol. Metab. [Internet] 2009 [cited 2020 Aug 9];94. Available from: https://pubmed.ncbi.nlm.nih.gov/19820013/

18. Gillespie AL, Calderwood D, Hobson L, Green BD. Whey proteins have beneficial effects on intestinal enteroendocrine cells stimulating cell growth and increasing the production and secretion of incretin hormones. Food Chem. [Internet] 2015 [cited 2020 Aug 9];189. Available from: https://pubmed.ncbi.nlm.nih.gov/26190610/

19. Foltz M, Ansems P, Schwarz J, Tasker MC, Lourbakos A, Gerhardt CC. Protein hydrolysates induce CCK release from enteroendocrine cells and act as partial agonists of the CCK1 receptor. J. Agric. Food Chem. [Internet] 2008 [cited 2020 Aug 9];56. Available from: https://pubmed.ncbi.nlm.nih.gov/18211011/

20. [No title] [Internet]. [cited 2020 Feb 24];Available from: http://www.fao.org/ag/humannutrition/36216-04a2f02ec02eafd4f457dd2c9851b4c45.pdf

21. pubmeddev, Sarwar Gilani G E al. Impact of antinutritional factors in food proteins on the digestibility of protein and the bioavailability of amino acids and on protein quality. - PubMed - NCBI [Internet]. [cited 2020 Feb 24];Available from: https://www.ncbi.nlm.nih.gov/pubmed/23107545

22. Examine.com. How much protein do you need per day? [Internet]. Examine.com2020 [cited 2020 Feb 24];Available from: https://examine.com/nutrition/how-much-protein-do-you-need/

23. pubmeddev, Mitchell CJ E al. Soy protein ingestion results in less prolonged p70S6 kinase phosphorylation compared to whey protein after resistance exercise in older men. - PubMed - NCBI [Internet]. [cited 2020 Feb 24];Available from: https://www.ncbi.nlm.nih.gov/pubmed/25674042

24. Rogerson D. Vegan diets: practical advice for athletes and exercisers. J. Int. Soc. Sports Nutr. 2017;14:36.

25. Blomstrand E, Eliasson J, Karlsson HKR, Köhnke R. Branched-Chain Amino Acids Activate Key Enzymes in Protein Synthesis after Physical Exercise [Internet]. The Journal of Nutrition2006;136:269S – 273S. Available from: http://dx.doi.org/10.1093/jn/136.1.269s

26. Norton LE, Wilson GJ, Layman DK, Moulton CJ, Garlick PJ. Leucine content of dietary proteins is a determinant of postprandial skeletal muscle protein synthesis in adult rats [Internet]. Nutrition & Metabolism2012;9:67. Available from: http://dx.doi.org/10.1186/1743-7075-9-67

27. Czajka A, Kania EM, Genovese L, Corbo A, Merone G, Luci C, et al. Daily oral supplementation with collagen peptides combined with vitamins and other bioactive compounds improves skin elasticity and has a beneficial effect on joint and general wellbeing [Internet]. Nutrition Research2018;57:97–108. Available from: http://dx.doi.org/10.1016/j.nutres.2018.06.001

28. Proksch E, Segger D, Degwert J, Schunck M, Zague V, Oesser S. Oral supplementation of specific collagen peptides has beneficial effects on human skin physiology: a double-blind, placebo-controlled study. Skin Pharmacol. Physiol. 2014;27:47–55.

29. Proksch E, Schunck M, Zague V, Segger D, Degwert J, Oesser S. Oral Intake of Specific Bioactive Collagen Peptides Reduces Skin Wrinkles and Increases Dermal Matrix Synthesis [Internet]. Skin Pharmacology and Physiology2014;27:113–9. Available from: http://dx.doi.org/10.1159/000355523

30. Zdzieblik D, Oesser S, Gollhofer A, König D. Improvement of activity-related knee joint discomfort following supplementation of specific collagen peptides. Appl. Physiol. Nutr. Metab. 2017;42:588–95.

31. König D, Oesser S, Scharla S, Zdzieblik D, Gollhofer A. Specific Collagen Peptides Improve Bone Mineral Density and Bone Markers in Postmenopausal Women-A Randomized Controlled Study. Nutrients [Internet] 2018;10. Available from: http://dx.doi.org/10.3390/nu10010097

32. Lopez HL, Ziegenfuss TN, Park J. Evaluation of the Effects of BioCell Collagen, a Novel Cartilage Extract, on Connective Tissue Support and Functional Recovery From Exercise. Integr. Med. 2015;14:30–8.

33. Phillips SM. Current Concepts and Unresolved Questions in Dietary Protein Requirements and Supplements in Adults. Front Nutr 2017;4:13.

34. Kawada C, Yoshida T, Yoshida H, Matsuoka R, Sakamoto W, Odanaka W, et al. Ingested hyaluronan moisturizes dry skin. Nutr. J. 2014;13:70.

35. Coletta JM, Bell SJ, Roman AS. Omega-3 Fatty acids and pregnancy. Rev. Obstet. Gynecol. 2010;3:163–71.

36. Tan SY. Effects of Different Dietary Fatty Acids on Human Energy Balance, Body Weight, Fat Mass, and Abdominal Fat [Internet]. Nutrition in the Prevention and Treatment of Abdominal Obesity2014;417–27. Available from: http://dx.doi.org/10.1016/b978-0-12-407869-7.00036-2

37. Huang CB, Ebersole JL. A novel bioactivity of omega-3 polyunsaturated fatty acids and their ester derivatives. Mol. Oral Microbiol. 2010;25:75–80.

38. Key Recommendations: Components of Healthy Eating Patterns - 2015-2020 Dietary Guidelines | health.gov [Internet]. [cited 2020 Apr 6];Available from: https://health.gov/our-work/food-nutrition/2015-2020-dietary-guidelines/guidelines/chapter-1/key-recommendations/

39. Micha R, Mozaffarian D. Trans fatty acids: effects on cardiometabolic health and implications for policy. Prostaglandins Leukot. Essent. Fatty Acids 2008;79:147–52.

40. Morton AM, Furtado JD, Mendivil CO, Sacks FM. Dietary unsaturated fat increases HDL metabolic pathways involving apoE favorable to reverse cholesterol transport [Internet]. JCI Insight2019;4. Available from: http://dx.doi.org/10.1172/jci.insight.124620

41. pubmeddev, Mandøe MJ E al. The 2-monoacylglycerol moiety of dietary fat appears to be responsible for the fat-induced release of GLP-1 in humans. - PubMed - NCBI [Internet]. [cited 2020 Feb 28];Available from: https://www.ncbi.nlm.nih.gov/pubmed/26178726

42. pubmeddev, Serrano P E al. Influence of type of dietary fat (olive and sunflower oil) upon gastric acid secretion and release of gastrin, somatostatin, and peptide YY in man. - PubMed - NCBI [Internet]. [cited 2020 Feb 28];Available from: https://www.ncbi.nlm.nih.gov/pubmed/9073149

43. pubmeddev, Gibbons C E al. Postprandial profiles of CCK after high fat and high carbohydrate meals and the relationship to satiety in humans. - PubMed - NCBI [Internet]. [cited 2020 Feb 28];Available from: https://www.ncbi.nlm.nih.gov/pubmed/26429068

44. pubmeddev, Kratz M E al. Dairy fat intake is associated with glucose tolerance, hepatic and systemic insulin sensitivity, and liver fat but not -cell function in humans. - PubMed - NCBI [Internet]. [cited 2020 Feb 28];Available from: https://www.ncbi.nlm.nih.gov/pubmed/24740208

45. pubmeddev, Casas-Agustench P E al. Effects of one serving of mixed nuts on serum lipids, insulin resistance and inflammatory markers in patients with the metabolic syndrome. - PubMed - NCBI [Internet]. [cited 2020 Feb 28]; Available from: https://www.ncbi.nlm.nih.gov/pubmed/20031380

46. pubmeddev, Lopez S E al. Effects of meals rich in either monounsaturated or saturated fat on lipid concentrations and on insulin secretion and action in subjects with high ... - PubMed - NCBI [Internet]. [cited 2020 Feb 28];Available from: https://www.ncbi.nlm.nih.gov/pubmed/21209225

47. Wang C, Catlin DH, Starcevic B, Heber D, Ambler C, Berman N, et al. Low-fat high-fiber diet decreased serum and urine androgens in men. J. Clin. Endocrinol. Metab. 2005;90:3550–9.

48. Erbsloh F, Klarner P, Bernsmeier A. [The balance of cerebral sugar metabolism]. Klin. Wochenschr. 1958;36:849–52.

49. Helge JW. Prolonged adaptation to fat-rich diet and training; effects on body fat stores and insulin resistance in man. Int. J. Obes. 2002;26:1118–24.

50. Jensen J, Rustad PI, Kolnes AJ, Lai Y-C. The Role of Skeletal Muscle Glycogen Breakdown for Regulation of Insulin Sensitivity by Exercise. Front. Physiol. [Internet] 2011 [cited 2020 Mar 25];2. Available from: https://www.ncbi.nlm.nih.gov/pmc/articles/PMC3248697/

51. Jensen J, Ruge T, Lai Y-C, Svensson MK, Eriksson JW. Effects of adrenaline on whole-body glucose metabolism and insulin-mediated regulation of glycogen synthase and PKB phosphorylation in human skeletal muscle. Metabolism 2011;60:215–26.

52. Kidd PM. Omega-3 DHA and EPA for cognition, behavior, and mood: clinical findings and structural-functional synergies with cell membrane phospholipids. Altern. Med. Rev. 2007;12:207–27.

53. Leveritt M, Abernethy PJ. Effects of Carbohydrate Restriction on Strength Performance [Internet]. The Journal of Strength and Conditioning Research1999;13:52. Available from: 2.0.co;2">http://dx.doi.org/10.1519/1533-4287(1999)013<0052:eocros>2.0.co;2

54. Horswill CA, Hickner RC, Scott JR, Costill DL, Gould D. Weight loss, dietary carbohydrate modifications, and high intensity, physical performance. Med. Sci. Sports Exerc. 1990;22:470–6.

55. Iraki J, Fitschen P, Espinar S, Helms E. Nutrition Recommendations for Bodybuilders in the Off-Season: A Narrative Review. Sports (Basel) [Internet] 2019;7. Available from: http://dx.doi.org/10.3390/sports7070154

56. Welsh JA, Sharma AJ, Grellinger L, Vos MB. Consumption of added sugars is decreasing in the United States. Am. J. Clin. Nutr. 2011;94:726–34.

57. Archer E. In Defense of Sugar: A Critique of Diet-Centrism [Internet]. Progress in Cardiovascular Diseases2018;61:10–9. Available from: http://dx.doi.org/10.1016/j.pcad.2018.04.007

58. Sylvetsky AC, Hiedacavage A, Shah N, Pokorney P, Baldauf S, Merrigan K, et al. From biology to behavior: a cross disciplinary seminar series surrounding added sugar and low calorie sweetener consumption [Internet]. Obesity Science & Practice2019;5:203–19. Available from: http://dx.doi.org/10.1002/osp4.334

59. Grundmann O, Yoon SL, Mason S, Smith K. Gastrointestinal symptom improvement from fiber, STW 5, peppermint oil, and probiotics use-Results from an online survey. Complement. Ther. Med. 2018;41:225–30.

60. Dahl WJ, Agro NC, Eliasson ÅM, Mialki KL, Olivera JD, Rusch CT, et al. Health Benefits of Fiber Fermentation. J. Am. Coll. Nutr. 2017;36:127–36.

61. Bertoia ML, Mukamal KJ, Cahill LE, Hou T, Ludwig DS, Mozaffarian D, et al. Correction: Changes in Intake of Fruits and Vegetables and Weight Change in United States Men and Women Followed for Up to 24 Years: Analysis from Three Prospective Cohort Studies. PLoS Med. 2016;13:e1001956.

62. Peter Holzer AF. Neuropeptides and the Microbiota-Gut-Brain Axis. Adv. Exp. Med. Biol. 2014;817:195.

63. Little TJ, Horowitz M, Feinle-Bisset C. Role of cholecystokinin in appetite control and body weight regulation. Obes. Rev. [Internet] 2005 [cited 2020 Aug 16];6. Available from: https://pubmed.ncbi.nlm.nih.gov/16246215/

64. Bourdon I, Olson B, Backus R, Richter BD, Davis PA, Schneeman BO. Beans, as a source of dietary fiber, increase cholecystokinin and apolipoprotein b48 response to test meals in men. J. Nutr. [Internet] 2001 [cited 2020 Aug 16];131. Available from: https://pubmed.ncbi.nlm.nih.gov/11340104/

65. Ye Z, Arumugam V, Haugabrooks E, Williamson P, Hendrich S. Soluble dietary fiber (Fibersol-2) decreased hunger and increased satiety hormones in humans when ingested with a meal. Nutr. Res. [Internet] 2015 [cited 2020 Aug 16];35. Available from: https://pubmed.ncbi.nlm.nih.gov/25823991/

66. Marcason W. Is there evidence to support the claim that a gluten-free diet should be used for weight loss? J. Am. Diet. Assoc. 2011;111:1786.

67. Smith E. High Fiber Foods: How To Lose Weight When On A High Fiber Diet. 2018.

68. FOOD AND AGRICULTURE ORGANIZATION OF THE UNITED NATIONS. State of Food Insecurity in the World 2014. 2015.

69. Fletcher RH, Fairfield KM. Vitamins for chronic disease prevention in adults: clinical applications. JAMA 2002;287:3127–9.

70. Dong J-Y, Xun P, He K, Qin L-Q. Magnesium intake and risk of type 2 diabetes: meta-analysis of prospective cohort studies. Diabetes Care 2011;34:2116–22.

71. Higdon J, Drake VJ. Evidence-Based Approach to Vitamins and Minerals: Health Benefits and Intake Recommendations. Thieme; 2011.

72. Bailey RL, West KP Jr, Black RE. The epidemiology of global micronutrient deficiencies. Ann. Nutr. Metab. 2015;66 Suppl 2:22–33.

73. Yokoi K, Konomi A. Iron deficiency without anaemia is a potential cause of fatigue: meta-analyses of randomised controlled trials and cross-sectional studies. Br. J. Nutr. 2017;117:1422–31.

74. Huskisson E, Maggini S, Ruf M. The role of vitamins and minerals in energy metabolism and well-being. J. Int. Med. Res. 2007;35:277–89.

75. Calton JB. Prevalence of micronutrient deficiency in popular diet plans. J. Int. Soc. Sports Nutr. 2010;7:1–9.

76. pubmeddev, G Engel M E al. Micronutrient Gaps in Three Commercial Weight-Loss Diet Plans. - PubMed - NCBI [Internet]. [cited 2020 Mar 8];Available from: https://www.ncbi.nlm.nih.gov/pubmed/29361684

77. Streit L, MS, RDN, LD. Micronutrients: Types, Functions, Benefits and More [Internet]. Healthline2018 [cited 2020 Apr 21]; Available from: https://www.healthline.com/nutrition/micronutrients

78. pubmeddev, Swinburn BA E al. The global obesity pandemic: shaped by global drivers and local environments. - PubMed - NCBI [Internet]. [cited 2020 Mar 1];Available from: https://www.ncbi.nlm.nih.gov/pubmed/21872749/

79. Villines Z. Body fat percentage chart: Women, men, and calculations [Internet]. Medical News Today2020 [cited 2020 Jun 24]; Available from: https://www.medicalnewstoday.com/articles/body-fat-percentage-chart

80. Heyward VH, Wagner DR. Applied Body Composition Assessment. Human Kinetics Publishers; 2004.

81. Helms ER, Aragon AA, Fitschen PJ. Evidence-based recommendations for natural bodybuilding contest preparation: nutrition and supplementation [Internet]. Journal of the International Society of Sports Nutrition2014;11. Available from: http://dx.doi.org/10.1186/1550-2783-11-20

82. Bandegan A, Courtney-Martin G, Rafii M, Pencharz PB, Lemon PW. Indicator Amino Acid-Derived Estimate of Dietary Protein Requirement for Male Bodybuilders on a Nontraining Day Is Several-Fold Greater than the Current Recommended Dietary Allowance. J. Nutr. 2017;147:850–7.

83. Appendix 7. Nutritional Goals for Age-Sex Groups Based on Dietary Reference Intakes and Dietary Guidelines Recommendations - 2015-2020 Dietary Guidelines | health.gov [Internet]. [cited 2020 Apr 6];Available from: https://health.gov/our-work/food-nutrition/2015-2020-dietary-guidelines/guidelines/appendix-7/#table-a7-1-daily-nutritional-goals-for-age-sex-groups-based-on-d

84. Josse AR, Atkinson SA, Tarnopolsky MA, Phillips SM. Increased Consumption of Dairy Foods and Protein during Diet- and Exercise-Induced Weight Loss Promotes Fat Mass Loss and Lean Mass Gain in Overweight and Obese Premenopausal Women. J. Nutr. 2011;141:1626–34.

85. Phillips SM. Dietary Protein: Minimal Requirements vs. Optimal Intake [Internet]. Medicine & Science in Sports & Exercise2008;40:72. Available from:

86. Alex Leaf JA. The Effects of Overfeeding on Body Composition: The Role of Macronutrient Composition – A Narrative Review. Int. J. Exerc. Sci. 2017;10:1275.

87. Volpi E. Is leucine content in dietary protein the key to muscle preservation in older women? Am. J. Clin. Nutr. 2018;107:143.

88. NHANES 2009-2010: Dietary Interview - Total Nutrient Intakes, First Day Data Documentation, Codebook, and Frequencies [Internet]. [cited 2020 Feb 21];Available from: https://wwwn.cdc.gov/Nchs/Nhanes/2009-2010/DR1TOT_F.htm#Component_Description

89. Key Recommendations: Components of Healthy Eating Patterns - 2015-2020 Dietary Guidelines | health.gov [Internet]. [cited 2020 Apr 6]. Available from: https://health.gov/our-work/food-nutrition/2015-2020-dietary-guidelines/guidelines/chapter-1/key-recommendations/

90. Gokulakrishnan K, Deepa M, Monickaraj F, Mohan V. Relationship of body fat with insulin resistance and cardiometabolic risk factors among normal glucose-tolerant subjects. J. Postgrad. Med. 2011;57:184–8.

91. Roberts BM, Helms ER, Trexler ET, Fitschen PJ. Nutritional Recommendations for Physique Athletes. J. Hum. Kinet. 2020;71:79.

92. Wilson GJ, Layman DK, Moulton CJ, Norton LE, Anthony TG, Proud CG, et al. Leucine or carbohydrate supplementation reduces AMPK and eEF2 phosphorylation and extends postprandial muscle protein synthesis in rats. Am. J. Physiol. Endocrinol. Metab. 2011;301:E1236–42.

93. McGlory C, Wardle SL, Macnaughton LS. Pattern of protein ingestion to maximise muscle protein synthesis after resistance exercise [Internet]. The Journal of Physiology2013;591:2969–70. Available from: http://dx.doi.org/10.1113/jphysiol.2013.256156

94. Mamerow MM, Mettler JA, English KL, Casperson SL, Arentson-Lantz E, Sheffield-Moore M, et al. Dietary protein distribution positively influences 24-h muscle protein synthesis in healthy adults. J. Nutr. 2014;144:876–80.

95. Bird SP, Tarpenning KM, Marino FE. Liquid carbohydrate/essential amino acid ingestion during a short-term bout of resistance exercise suppresses myofibrillar protein degradation. Metabolism 2006;55:570–7.

96. Tipton KD. Role of protein and hydrolysates before exercise. Int. J. Sport Nutr. Exerc. Metab. 2007;17 Suppl:S77–86.

97. Foster RK, Marriott HE. Alcohol consumption in the new millennium ? weighing up the risks and benefits for our health [Internet]. Nutrition Bulletin2006;31:286–331. Available from: http://dx.doi.org/10.1111/j.1467-3010.2006.00588.x

98. Thomson CA, Wertheim BC, Hingle M, Wang L, Neuhouser ML, Gong Z, et al. Alcohol consumption and body weight change in postmenopausal women: results from the Women's Health Initiative. Int. J. Obes. 2012;36:1158–64.

99. Linardon J, Messer M, Fuller-Tyszkiewicz M. Meta-analysis of the effects of cognitive-behavioral therapy for binge-eating-type disorders on abstinence rates in nonrandomized effectiveness studies: Comparable outcomes to randomized, controlled trials? Int. J. Eat. Disord. 2018;51:1303–11.

100. Meule A, Westenhöfer J, Kübler A. Food cravings mediate the relationship between rigid, but not flexible control of eating behavior and dieting success. Appetite 2011;57:582–4.

101. Westenhoefer J, Engel D, Holst C, Lorenz J, Peacock M, Stubbs J, et al. Cognitive and weight-related correlates of flexible and rigid restrained eating behaviour. Eat. Behav. 2013;14:69–72.

117. Lorente-Cebrián S, Costa AGV, Navas-Carretero S, Zabala M, Alfredo Martínez J, Moreno-Aliaga MJ. Role of omega-3 fatty acids in obesity, metabolic syndrome, and cardiovascular diseases: a review of the evidence [Internet]. Journal of Physiology and Biochemistry2013;69:633–51. Available from: http://dx.doi.org/10.1007/s13105-013-0265-4

118. Authority EFS, European Food Safety Authority. Outcome of the Public consultation on the Draft Opinion of the Scientific Panel on Dietetic Products, Nutrition, and Allergies (NDA) on Dietary Reference Values for fats, including saturated fatty acids, polyunsaturated fatty acids, monounsaturated fatty acids, trans fatty acids, and cholesterol [Internet]. EFSA Journal2010;8. Available from: http://dx.doi.org/10.2903/j.efsa.2010.1507

119. Sekikawa A, David Curb J, Ueshima H, El-Saed A, Kadowaki T, Abbott RD, et al. Marine-Derived n-3 Fatty Acids and Atherosclerosis in Japanese, Japanese-American, and White Men [Internet]. Journal of the American College of Cardiology2008;52:417–24. Available from: http://dx.doi.org/10.1016/j.jacc.2008.03.047

120. Zhang J, Sasaki S, Amano K, Kesteloot H. Fish consumption and mortality from all causes, ischemic heart disease, and stroke: an ecological study. Prev. Med. 1999;28:520–9.

121. Gomez J. Omega-3 Continues to Show Protection Against Heart Disease-Related Death Without Prostate Cancer Risk [Internet]. [cited 2020 Oct 7];Available from: https://intermountainhealthcare.org/news/2019/11/omega-3-continues-to-show-protection-against-heart-disease-related-death-without-prostate-cancer-risk/

122. Al Khatib HK, Harding SV, Darzi J, Pot GK. The effects of partial sleep deprivation on energy balance: a systematic review and meta-analysis. Eur. J. Clin. Nutr. 2016;71:614–24.

123. Andersen LP, Rosenberg J, Gögenur I. Perioperative melatonin: not ready for prime time. Br. J. Anaesth. [Internet] 2014 [cited 2020 Oct 7];112. Available from: https://pubmed.ncbi.nlm.nih.gov/24318695/

124. Burke LM. Caffeine and sports performance [Internet]. Applied Physiology, Nutrition, and Metabolism2008;33:1319–34. Available from: http://dx.doi.org/10.1139/h08-130

125. Kurobe K, Nakao S, Nishiwaki M, Matsumoto N. Combined effect of coffee ingestion and repeated bouts of low-intensity exercise on fat oxidation. Clin. Physiol. Funct. Imaging 2017;37:148–54.

126. Harpaz E, Tamir S, Weinstein A, Weinstein Y. The effect of caffeine on energy balance. J. Basic Clin. Physiol. Pharmacol. 2017;28:1–10.

127. Belza A, Toubro S, Astrup A. The effect of caffeine, green tea and tyrosine on thermogenesis and energy intake. Eur. J. Clin. Nutr. 2009;63:57–64.

128. Acheson KJ, Zahorska-Markiewicz B, Pittet P, Anantharaman K, Jéquier E. Caffeine and coffee: their influence on metabolic rate and substrate utilization in normal weight and obese individuals. Am. J. Clin. Nutr. 1980;33:989–97.

129. Davoodi SH, Hajimiresmaiel SJ, Ajami M, Mohseni-Bandpei A, Ayatollahi SA, Dowlatshahi K, et al. Caffeine treatment prevented from weight regain after calorie shifting diet induced weight loss. Iran J Pharm Res 2014;13:707–18.

130. Brooks JH, Wyld K. Caffeine Supplementation as an Ergogenic Aid for Muscular Strength and Endurance: A Recommendation for Coaches and Athletes [Internet]. Journal of Athletic Enhancement2016;5. Available from: http://dx.doi.org/10.4172/2324-9080.1000235

131. Goldstein E, Jacobs PL, Whitehurst M, Penhollow T, Antonio J. Caffeine enhances upper body strength in resistance trained women. J. Int. Soc. Sports Nutr. 2010;7:18.

132. Dulloo AG, Duret C, Rohrer D, Girardier L, Mensi N, Fathi M, et al. Efficacy of a green tea extract rich in catechin polyphenols and caffeine in increasing 24-h energy expenditure and fat oxidation in humans [Internet]. The American Journal of Clinical Nutrition1999;70:1040–5. Available from: http://dx.doi.org/10.1093/ajcn/70.6.1040

133. Ostojic SM. Yohimbine: the effects on body composition and exercise performance in soccer players. Res. Sports Med. 2006;14:289–99.

134. Lafontan M, Berlan M, Galitzky J, Montastruc JL. Alpha-2 adrenoceptors in lipolysis: 2 antagonists and lipid-mobilizing strategies [Internet]. The American Journal of Clinical Nutrition1992;55:219S – 227S. Available from: http://dx.doi.org/10.1093/ajcn/55.1.219s

135. Creatine [Internet]. [cited 2020 Oct 7];Available from: https://my.clevelandclinic.org/health/drugs/17674-creatine

136. Mihic S, MacDONALD JR, McKENZIE S, Tarnopolsky MA. Acute creatine loading increases fat-free mass, but does not affect blood pressure, plasma creatinine, or CK activity in men and women [Internet]. Medicine & Science in Sports & Exercise2000;32:291. Available from: http://dx.doi.org/10.1097/00005768-200002000-00007

137. Bemben MG, Lamont HS. Creatine Supplementation and Exercise Performance [Internet]. Sports Medicine2005;35:107–25. Available from: http://dx.doi.org/10.2165/00007256-200535020-00002

138. Candow DG, Chilibeck PD, Forbes SC. Creatine supplementation and aging musculoskeletal health. Endocrine 2014;45:354–61.

139. Roitman S, Green T, Osher Y, Karni N, Levine J. Creatine monohydrate in resistant depression: a preliminary study. Bipolar Disord. 2007;9:754–8.

140. Beal MF. Neuroprotective effects of creatine. Amino Acids 2011;40:1305–13.

141. Buford TW, Kreider RB, Stout JR, Greenwood M, Campbell B, Spano M, et al. International Society of Sports Nutrition position stand: creatine supplementation and exercise. J. Int. Soc. Sports Nutr. 2007;4:6.

142. Kreider RB, Peter Jung Y. Creatine supplementation in exercise, sport, and medicine [Internet]. The Journal of Exercise Nutrition and Biochemistry2011;6:53–69. Available from: http://dx.doi.org/10.5717/jenb.2011.15.2.53

143. Dalton RL, Sowinski RJ, Grubic TJ, Collins PB, Coletta AM, Reyes AG, et al. Hematological and Hemodynamic Responses to Acute and Short-Term Creatine Nitrate Supplementation. Nutrients [Internet] 2017;9. Available from: http://dx.doi.org/10.3390/nu9121359

144. Saunders B, Elliott-Sale K, Artioli GG, Swinton PA, Dolan E, Roschel H, et al. -alanine supplementation to improve exercise capacity and performance: a systematic review and meta-analysis. Br. J. Sports Med. 2017;51:658–69.

145. Bailey SJ, Blackwell JR, Lord T, Vanhatalo A, Winyard PG, Jones AM. l-Citrulline supplementation improves O2 uptake kinetics and high-intensity exercise performance in humans [Internet]. Journal of Applied Physiology 2015;119:385–95. Available from: http://dx.doi.org/10.1152/japplphysiol.00192.2014

146. Bendahan D, Mattei JP, Ghattas B, Confort-Gouny S, Le Guern ME, Cozzone PJ. Citrulline/malate promotes aerobic energy production in human exercising muscle. Br. J. Sports Med. 2002;36:282–9.

147. Figueroa A, Wong A, Jaime SJ, Gonzales JU. Influence of L-citrulline and watermelon supplementation on vascular function and exercise performance. Curr. Opin. Clin. Nutr. Metab. Care 2017;20:92–8.

148. Pérez-Guisado J, Jakeman PM. Citrulline Malate Enhances Athletic Anaerobic Performance and Relieves Muscle Soreness [Internet]. Journal of Strength and Conditioning Research 2010;24:1215–22. Available from: http://dx.doi.org/10.1519/jsc.0b013e3181cb28e0

149. Allerton TD, Proctor DN, Stephens JM, Dugas TR, Spielmann G, Irving BA. l-Citrulline Supplementation: Impact on Cardiometabolic Health. Nutrients [Internet] 2018 [cited 2020 Oct 5];10. Available from: https://www.ncbi.nlm.nih.gov/pmc/articles/PMC6073798/

150. Miller PE, Perez V. Low-calorie sweeteners and body weight and composition: a meta-analysis of randomized controlled trials and prospective cohort studies [Internet]. The American Journal of Clinical Nutrition 2014;100:765–77. Available from: http://dx.doi.org/10.3945/ajcn.113.082826

151. Peters JC, Wyatt HR, Foster GD, Pan Z, Wojtanowski AC, Vander Veur SS, et al. The effects of water and non-nutritive sweetened beverages on weight loss during a 12-week weight loss treatment program. Obesity 2014;22:1415–21.

152. Peters JC, Beck J, Cardel M, Wyatt HR, Foster GD, Pan Z, et al. The effects of water and non-nutritive sweetened beverages on weight loss and weight maintenance: A randomized clinical trial. Obesity 2016;24:297–304.

153. Bleich SN, Wolfson JA, Vine S, Wang YC. Diet-beverage consumption and caloric intake among US adults, overall and by body weight. Am. J. Public Health 2014;104:e72–8.

154. Ruanpeng D, Thongprayoon C, Cheungpasitporn W, Harindhanavudhi T. Sugar and artificially sweetened beverages linked to obesity: a systematic review and meta-analysis. QJM 2017;110:513–20.

155. Campos V, Despland C, Brandejsky V, Kreis R, Schneiter P, Chiolero A, et al. Sugar- and artificially sweetened beverages and intrahepatic fat: A randomized controlled trial. Obesity [Internet] 2015 [cited 2020 Aug 29];23. Available from: https://pubmed.ncbi.nlm.nih.gov/26727115/

156. Sugar-sweetened beverage, diet soda, and fatty liver disease in the Framingham Heart Study cohorts. J. Hepatol. 2015;63:462–9.

157. Cuomo R, Sarnelli G, Savarese MF, Buyckx M. Carbonated beverages and gastrointestinal system: between myth and reality. Nutr. Metab. Cardiovasc. Dis. [Internet] 2009 [cited 2020 Aug 29];19. Available from: https://pubmed.ncbi.nlm.nih.gov/19502016/

158. Johnson T, Gerson L, Hershcovici T, Stave C, Fass R. Systematic review: the effects of carbonated beverages on gastro-oesophageal reflux disease. Aliment. Pharmacol. Ther. [Internet] 2010 [cited 2020 Aug 29];31. Available from: https://pubmed.ncbi.nlm.nih.gov/20055784/

159. Cuomo R, Andreozzi P, Zito FP. Alcoholic beverages and carbonated soft drinks: consumption and gastrointestinal cancer risks. Cancer Treat. Res. [Internet] 2014 [cited 2020 Aug 29];159. Available from: https://pubmed.ncbi.nlm.nih.gov/24114477/

160. Lohner S, Toews I, Meerpohl JJ. Health outcomes of non-nutritive sweeteners: analysis of the research landscape. Nutr. J. 2017;16:55.

161. Nettleton JE, Reimer RA, Shearer J. Reshaping the gut microbiota: Impact of low calorie sweeteners and the link to insulin resistance? Physiol. Behav. [Internet] 2016 [cited 2020 Aug 29];164. Available from: https://pubmed.ncbi.nlm.nih.gov/27090230/

162. Suez J, Korem T, Zilberman-Schapira G, Segal E, Elinav E. Non-caloric artificial sweeteners and the microbiome: findings and challenges. Gut Microbes [Internet] 2015 [cited 2020 Aug 29];6. Available from: https://pubmed.ncbi.nlm.nih.gov/25831243/

163. Al-Goblan AS, Al-Alfi MA, Khan MZ. Mechanism linking diabetes mellitus and obesity. Diabetes Metab. Syndr. Obes. 2014;7:587–91.

164. Center for Food Safety, Nutrition A. Additional Information about High-Intensity Sweeteners [Internet]. 2020 [cited 2020 Aug 30]; Available from: https://www.fda.gov/food/food-additives-petitions/additional-information-about-high-intensity-sweeteners-permitted-use-food-united-states

165. Bordoni A, Danesi F, Dardevet D, Dupont D, Fernandez AS, Gille D, et al. Dairy products and inflammation: A review of the clinical evidence. Crit. Rev. Food Sci. Nutr. [Internet] 2017 [cited 2020 Sep 4];57. Available from: https://pubmed.ncbi.nlm.nih.gov/26287637/

166. Dougkas A, Reynolds CK, Givens ID, Elwood PC, Minihane AM. Associations between dairy consumption and body weight: a review of the evidence and underlying mechanisms. Nutr. Res. Rev. 2011;24:72–95.

167. Website [Internet]. [cited 2020 Aug 27];Available from: https://www.researchgate.net/publication/51508091_Increased_Consumption_of_Dairy_Foods_and_Protein_during_Diet-_and_Exercise-Induced_Weight_Loss_Promotes_Fat_Mass_Loss_and_Lean_Mass_Gain_in_Overweight_and_Obese_Premenopausal_Women

168. Panahi S, Tremblay A. The Potential Role of Yogurt in Weight Management and Prevention of Type 2 Diabetes [Internet]. Journal of the American College of Nutrition2016;35:717–31. Available from: http://dx.doi.org/10.1080/07315724.2015.1102103

169. Jones AL. The Gluten-Free Diet: Fad or Necessity? Diabetes Spectr. 2017;30:118.

170. M U Yang TBVI. Composition of weight lost during short-term weight reduction. Metabolic responses of obese subjects to starvation and l low-calorie ketogenic and nonketogenic diets. J. Clin. Invest. 1976;58:722.

171. Masood W, Annamaraju P, Uppaluri KR. Ketogenic Diet. In: StatPearls [Internet]. StatPearls Publishing; 2020.

172. Kirkpatrick CF, Bolick JP, Kris-Etherton PM, Sikand G, Aspry KE, Soffer DE, et al. Review of current evidence and clinical recommendations on the effects of low-carbohydrate and very-low-carbohydrate (including ketogenic) diets for the management of body weight and other cardiometabolic risk factors: A scientific statement from the National Lipid Association Nutrition and Lifestyle Task Force [Internet]. Journal of Clinical Lipidology2019;13:689–711.e1. Available from: http://dx.doi.org/10.1016/j.jacl.2019.08.003